Beat Insomnia with NLP

For my brother, Aleister.

Teach®
Yourself

Beat Insomnia with NLP

Adrian Tannock

First published in Great Britain in 2011 by Hodder Education. An Hachette UK company.

First published in US in 2011 by The McGraw-Hill Companies, Inc.

This edition published in 2018 by John Murray Learning.

Copyright © Adrian Tannock 2011, 2018

British Library Cataloguing in Publication Data: a catalogue record for this title is available from the British Library.

Library of Congress Catalog Card Number: on file.

ISBN: 978 1 473 67935 1

eISBN: 978 1 473 67936 8

1

Typeset by Cenveo® Publisher Services.

Printed and bound in Great Britain by CPI Group (UK) Ltd., Croydon, CR0 4YY.

John Murray Learning policy is to use papers that are natural, renewable and recyclable products and made from wood grown in sustainable forests. The logging and manufacturing processes are expected to conform to the environmental regulations of the country of origin.

Carmelite House
50 Victoria Embankment
London EC4Y 0DZ
www.hodder.co.uk

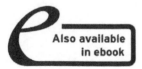

Also available in ebook

Acknowledgements

I would like to thank the following people for their help and encouragement in writing this book: Kerry Foster, Mate Mićovanis, Hannah Gray and Victoria Roddam.

Contents

Meet the author

For years I have been helping people overcome their difficulties with insomnia. I start by teaching people how sleep works, and then focus on putting in place simple but effective changes to their daily lives. For some, this simply means changing certain habits to be more sleep-promoting. For others: fears, anxieties and limiting beliefs need to change before sleep can improve.

There are many reasons why people find it difficult to sleep. To help as many of my clients as possible, I have researched (and implemented) different approaches to beating insomnia and sleeping soundly. The most effective method, I have found, has been to augment established approaches with specific relaxation and visualization techniques drawn from the field of Neuro-linguistic Programming (NLP). This book is designed to guide you through a programme of change, just as if we were working together in person.

In my work, both as therapist and author, I have been determined to help people find freedom in their lives: freedom from restriction, from frustration and from pain. Insomnia can cause untold misery, and here I hope to help you find the freedom that you are looking for. My approach is simple and light-hearted but also thorough and effective. Beating insomnia will change your life. Take care, take your time, and you have every chance of success. With that thought in mind, let's make a start.

In one minute

Sleep is driven by two independent bodily processes: the *circadian* process, responsible for the timing of sleep, and the *homeostatic* process, responsible for the intensity of sleep. When something goes wrong with one (or both) of these processes, sleep disorders may develop. The most common sleep disorder is insomnia: a major public health problem consisting of sleeplessness, frustration, anxiety, fatigue and eventually exhaustion.

NLP stands for Neuro-linguistic Programming. It is a collection of ideas and mental techniques gathered together in order to bring about positive change. NLP can help people overcome insomnia by achieving the following: making it easier to implement good sleep hygiene (a collection of improvements designed to promote sleep), alleviating anxious thoughts and feelings, helping people feel drowsy, relaxed and ready to sleep, and restoring confidence in their ability to sleep.

Relaxation also helps. Insomnia can be challenged by learning to relax your body while breathing slowly and deeply. Once relaxed in this way, a person can bring feelings of sleepiness flooding back, or use their imaginations to go on a relaxing journey in their minds. In such states we can program ourselves to be free from fear, pain or limiting belief. Our beliefs can either detract from our chances of sleep, or enhance them.

Learning how to overcome insomnia can take practice, and determination, but you can beat it. Overcome insomnia, and you are learning how to take control of yourself, and your life.

1

Understanding insomnia

In this chapter you will learn:
- *about the basics of sleep*
- *how to tell if you have insomnia*
- *about the different types of insomnia*
- *about other sleep disorders.*

> *O sleep! O gentle sleep!*
> *Nature's soft nurse, how have I frighted thee,*
> *That thou no more wilt weigh my eyelids down*
> *And steep my senses in forgetfulness?*

William Shakespeare

In times such as these, how valuable is sleep? In our increasingly 24-hour society, it is the timekeeping of modern life that dictates how we work and rest. Our biological clocks, honed by many millions of years of evolution, are struggling to keep up. Perhaps unsurprisingly, it is estimated that around 10–15 per cent of the UK population experiences chronic insomnia. It is a major public health problem with serious consequences. Left unchecked, insomnia can be a miserable experience.

This book has been written to guide you towards better sleep. It will be a straightforward process, and a gentle one. Some of the recommendations in this book will be easy to implement. Others will be challenging at first, getting easier with practice or time. Despite the pressures of modern life, we retain a natural ability to sleep. This book will reconnect you with that ability.

What to expect

To begin, we will learn about sleep and sleeplessness, Neuro-linguistic Programming (NLP) and how it is best implemented. In Chapter 4 we will discuss your sleeping environment, and put in place changes that will make it ideal for sleep.

From there we will optimize your behaviours, your thoughts and your feelings so they are sleep-promoting. Each recommendation will be explained thoroughly. We will work out ways to help you sleep more easily. In order for you to find the change you are looking for, to enjoy a more refreshing and restorative sleep, our approach will be simple and collaborative.

Towards the end of this book we will turn our attention to any outstanding difficulties, ironing out any problems that remain. It may take four weeks or so before you fully complete the programme laid out in this book, and then a little while longer as you fine-tune it to suit your lifestyle. Within two months or so, your ability to sleep will be greatly improved. You will feel that you have turned a corner, your troubles with sleep left behind. After three months, these changes will be fixed firmly in place and you will begin to see yourself as somebody who can sleep easily and naturally.

Many people will find that simply reading this book will aid sleep. Contained within its pages are powerful suggestions designed to promote sleep. As we work through this comprehensive programme together, focus on practising the exercises repeatedly. As a result, your sleep will improve.

The basics of sleep

So, what is sleep? And why do we need it? For the most part, when we sleep, we are physically inactive. We lose awareness of ourselves and of our environment. Sleep unfolds in cycles, typically four or five cycles per night, where we alternate between periods of *deep sleep*, followed by shorter periods of *Rapid Eye Movement (REM) sleep*. During the first part of the night there tends to be more deep sleep, and during the second part of the night we experience longer periods of REM sleep.

The deep sleep period of each cycle comprises four stages. Stage 1 is in fact very light sleep, coming just after wakefulness. Stage 2 then quickly follows as our muscles relax, and our heart rate and breathing slows. From there, a person phases into much deeper sleep, Stages 3 and 4, where our breathing and heart rate slow further. It is during this deeper sleep that restorative processes in the body take place. Stages 3 and 4 are known as *slow-wave sleep*, because brain activity during this period is markedly different from when we are awake. One sleep cycle, from Stage 1 sleep through to slow-wave sleep and then REM sleep, can take around 90 minutes or so.

As we approach the end of each cycle, we enter REM sleep, which is characterized by the jerky rapid eye movements that give it its name. The onset of REM sleep is abrupt, and in some ways our brain activity is similar to when we are awake. REM sleep is when most of our dreaming occurs. Usually, there is a complete paralysis of our body, most likely to stop us from acting out our dreams. Periods of REM sleep become longer in duration as the night progresses. This is why people tend to remember the dreams they have in the early morning hours, rather than those dreams that happen in the dead of night.

So, there are periods of restorative slow-wave sleep, followed by short bursts of REM sleep. As the night progresses, the duration and intensity of the slow-wave sleep cycle reduces, and REM sleep becomes more prevalent. Usually a person will wake several times each night. However, these awakenings are rarely noticed or remembered, except in cases of insomnia.

Insight – the need for sleep

We spend around a third of our lives asleep. It is essential to brain function, and losing sleep can result in consequences for our mood, our cognitive ability and our body's ability to restore itself. A loss of sleep also affects our ability to learn and remember, and can affect our immune system. Those of us who lose sleep regularly will frequently report a dissatisfaction with life.

These days, a great deal is understood about the nature of sleep. Typically, each night, we get about three to four hours of slow-wave sleep. It is estimated that around two hours of deep, slow-wave sleep is required for our body to remain healthy.

The majority of people will sleep for between seven and eight hours per night. However, there is no standard amount of sleep we, as humans, require. The amount of sleep you need is simply the length of time it takes for you to function normally on the following day. That might be six hours or it might be nine hours. There is no prescribed length of time that suits all people; our needs are unique to us.

We do tend to need less sleep as we grow older. For example, there is a strong relationship between sleep and the body's production of growth hormone. In our adult life the production of growth hormone reduces markedly, therefore we require less sleep. As the amount of slow-wave sleep we get decreases, our sleep becomes increasingly fragmented. The relationship between sleep and our body is complex. It is driven by two independent processes: the *circadian* process and the *homeostatic* process.

THE CIRCADIAN PROCESS

Circadian (from Latin, meaning 'around a day') rhythms are bodily cycles that repeat once per day, and which regulate the daily function of our body and brain. Most circadian rhythms are driven by our master body clock, and are responsible for processes such as liver function, body temperature, hormone release and our sleep–wake cycle. Each night the circadian process sends signals to the body that induce sleep. By 4 a.m. this circadian-based drive to sleep is at its strongest. By mid-morning the next day, the circadian process will have replaced sleep-promoting signals with wakefulness-promoting signals, keeping us alert during the day. This cycle of sleep-promotion and wakefulness-promotion continues day after day, and is independent of tiredness or the amount of sleep we get.

The circadian process is dependent on our internal body clock. This clock is in fact a pair of pinhead-sized structures found in the hypothalamus region of the brain. This part of the brain is connected to our eyes, and is sensitive to light. Generally, exposing yourself to daylight during the early hours of the day helps to set your body clock for an earlier rise time. Other external cues, such as keeping to a regular time for eating, working, exercising and socializing, also regulate our body's internal clock. It is telling that people with insomnia often struggle to keep to a regular schedule, frequently skipping breakfast or rising at different times each morning. An irregular schedule further weakens the ticking of our body clock, making sleep even more problematic in future. Sleep is very much dependent on timing; it is the circadian process that regulates the *timing* of sleep.

THE HOMEOSTATIC PROCESS

Homeostasis means a tendency towards balance. In this context, the homeostatic process is designed to regulate the balance between time spent awake and time spent asleep. To achieve this, the body creates a pressure to sleep that increases with each hour awake. This pressure to sleep usually peaks at around 16 hours after waking up in the morning.

Homeostatic sleep pressure diminishes when asleep. If we sleep well during the night, our drive to sleep is satisfied upon waking the next day. When our sleep is poor or fractured, we are then left with a *sleep debt*: our sleep drive hasn't been satisfied and we feel tired and run down. This increased sleep pressure, in theory, means we will sleep more deeply during the next night. The homeostatic process controls the *intensity* of sleep.

When working well, it is an effective system. The circadian process and the homeostatic process operate in concert so both systems promote the onset of sleep at the same time. There is a correlation between the pressure generated by the homeostatic process and the intensity of slow-wave activity found in the brain during sleep. Remember, it is during Stages 3 and 4 slow-wave sleep that our body's restorative processes take place. Our body's drive to sleep is more focused on achieving an intensely deep sleep, rather than simply sleeping for a fixed amount of time. This is important to remember.

So it's about timing and intensity. As with all complex systems, things can go wrong. For example, body clocks differ from person to person. For some of us, known as *larks*, getting up early (and going to bed early) suits best. For others, known as *owls*, early starts are difficult but staying awake, well into the early hours, feels very natural. Those of us who are *owls* can struggle with sleep deprivation because staying up late can clash with work commitments. Modern life often demands an early start.

Insight – tips for owls

Even in the case of *owls*, our body clocks can be made more compatible with our lives. As we mentioned earlier, keeping a regular time for rising, eating and socializing will keep our body clock ticking over nicely; our body clock synchronizes to environmental cues. As humans, we are nothing if not flexible.

For *owls*, the best thing to do is seek out sunlight in the early morning. If you live in the UK, this can be problematic to say the least! Sun lamps are not expensive, and can be an excellent tool for setting your body clock to be more compatible with early starts.

Irregular rising times also cause problems. Here, because we have not slept enough during the night, our drive to sleep compels us to spend extra time in bed. Although this satisfies the homeostatic drive (for an increased amount of slow-wave sleep), it wreaks havoc with our body clock, stressing our body and creating problems that then further interfere with our sleep–wake cycle. Sleep can be a fragile system, particularly for sufferers of insomnia.

Daytime naps, going to bed earlier than usual, sleeping in or cancelling activities because you feel tired all interfere with the circadian process (timing), and the homeostatic process (sleep pressure). Our work together will focus on strengthening these systems; synchronizing them so they each play their part in consistent and restorative sleep.

So, let's summarize what we have learned so far:

▶ Sleep unfolds in cycles, typically four or five cycles per night, where we alternate between deep sleep and REM sleep.
▶ Deep sleep unfolds over four stages. The first two stages are characterized by increased physical relaxation. Stages 3 and 4 are known as slow-wave sleep due to the slow nature of brain activity present during these stages.
▶ It is during slow-wave sleep that the body's natural restorative processes occur.
▶ As the night progresses, the duration and intensity of slow-wave sleep gives way to lengthier periods of REM sleep.
▶ Our sleep system is governed by two processes. One, the circadian process, is controlled by our body clock, and is responsible for the timing of sleep.
▶ The other, the homeostatic process, is wake-dependent, and is responsible for the intensity of slow-wave sleep we get each night.
▶ These two independent systems work together to help us fall asleep naturally.
▶ An irregular lifestyle will create an irregular body clock, which makes it difficult to sleep.
▶ Sleeping when we perhaps should be awake, for example sleeping in in the morning, weakens the homeostatic drive to sleep, also causing problems.

If you are reading this book, there is a good chance that you are having problems with your sleep. Now that we know what sleep is and how it works, let's take a look at those things that can go wrong. We will start with insomnia, the most commonly diagnosed sleep disorder. From there we'll take a look at the causes of insomnia, and how it can coexist with other medical or psychological conditions. Finally, we will consider other common sleep disorders, with advice as to what can be done in those cases.

How to tell if you have insomnia

Insomnia is defined as a difficulty in falling asleep, known as *sleep onset insomnia*, or difficulties in staying asleep or early morning wakening, both of which are known as *sleep maintenance insomnia*. Insomnia is usually caused by a failure of the sleep-promoting mechanisms described earlier in this chapter, most usually because these mechanisms are being overridden by alertness; for example, due to anxiety or pain.

Most people will experience insomnia at some stage in their life. *Transient insomnia* typically lasts for one or two nights, and usually occurs in response to a stressful event in life. This can include relatively minor events such as an argument with one's boss at work or receiving bad news. Often, we will experience transient insomnia before a big day; for example, wedding-night nerves. How many times have you been told, 'You've got a big day tomorrow! Get some sleep.'? The anxiety this thought can create then makes it more difficult to sleep. Focusing on the need to sleep is often a key component of insomnia.

Usually such problems or events blow over, and a person's sleep processes return to normal. When sleeplessness continues beyond a few days, it is termed *short-term insomnia*. Typically lasting anywhere up to several weeks, short-term insomnia is often connected with an ongoing event in a person's life. An impending redundancy, family troubles, a health scare – such events can cause sleepless nights; anxiety overrides our sleep processes and we lie awake tossing and turning. Again, as these difficulties subside, normal sleeping patterns typically return.

Jargon buster – the different types of insomnia

There are two different types of insomnia:

▶ *Primary insomnia*. This is where insomnia exists on its own.
▶ *Secondary insomnia*. This is where insomnia coexists with a medical or psychological condition.

There are two ways in which we can experience insomnia:

▶ *Sleep onset insomnia*. This refers to difficulties when trying to fall asleep.
▶ *Sleep maintenance insomnia*. This refers to difficulties in staying asleep: either waking up during the night or waking up too early in the morning.

Insomnia is divided into three different categories, depending on how long it is experienced for:

▶ *Transient insomnia*. This refers to insomnia which lasts no more than a day or two.
▶ *Short-term insomnia*. Typically, short-term insomnia will last for anywhere up to a couple of weeks.
▶ *Chronic insomnia*. This refers to insomnia that has really taken hold, and has lasted for more than a month.

There is a danger that short-term insomnia can *take hold*. If a person experiences insomnia for more than a month, they are suffering with *chronic insomnia*. This type of insomnia is unlikely to just work itself out. Left unchecked, chronic insomnia can last for years, even when the problems that caused it have long since passed. In such cases, some kind of action is required; for example, following the exercises and recommendations in this book.

In addition to difficulties falling asleep, staying asleep, or consistently waking up too early, there are some daytime factors to consider. Insomnia causes fatigue, concentration problems and a tendency towards frustration or irritability. There may be difficulties in coping with work or at home; sufferers may experience feeling run down. People with insomnia may start to fear bedtime, worrying about the effect sleeplessness is having on their lives. These worries can grip a person's mind, leading to obsessive thinking, anxiety and even depression. Finally, insomnia sufferers tend to fall into the trap of sleep-incompatible behaviours such as lying in bed awake night after night, which then makes matters worse, as we shall see.

THE DIFFERENCE BETWEEN FATIGUE AND SLEEPINESS

It is very important to note that daytime sleepiness is rarely a feature of insomnia. Insomnia sufferers are likely to feel fatigued, achy, irritable and so on, but these things do not cause people to fall asleep. There is a difference between feeling fatigued and sleepy. Fatigue is unpleasant. It will often leave you feeling that your daytime performance is impaired. You might yearn for sleep, and may be fixated on sleep or on how tired you feel. However, unless you are on the verge of nodding off during the day (or actually falling asleep), you are fatigued, rather than sleepy.

If daytime sleepiness is frequently present, that could indicate a problem known as *delayed sleep phase syndrome (DSPS)* – a circadian rhythm sleep disorder which we will discuss briefly later in this chapter.

Insomnia causes sleeplessness: sleeplessness combined with worry, frustration, fatigue, anxiety, and eventually, exhaustion. A person can inhabit a kind of twilight world, never feeling properly asleep or properly awake. There may be a tendency to take naps, which reduces one's drive to sleep and exacerbates the problem further. As we have mentioned, there can be a difficulty in coping. Work performance can suffer or friends and family can find it difficult to understand. Insomnia is a major problem which can have far-reaching consequences in a person's life.

Insomnia can play tricks on our mind. For example, our experience of time is relative. When lying in bed, awake, with little sensory input and a growing sense of tiredness and frustration, time seems to go by very slowly. Our subjective experience of insomnia can leave us feeling that we haven't slept a wink all night. And, yet, people with insomnia do sleep, it is just that their sleep is truncated to some extent. It can be quite difficult to overcome this *sleep misperception,* and later in this chapter we will introduce a tool that will help.

So, insomnia is not just sleeplessness:

▶ Insomnia can involve difficulty falling asleep, difficulty staying asleep or early morning wakening.

- ▶ During the day, insomnia can lead to frustration, anxiety, fatigue, impaired performance and exhaustion.
- ▶ Insomnia is usually caused by some kind of difficulty or stress in life. Most frequently, when the difficulty or stress has passed, sleeping patterns return to normal.
- ▶ Where insomnia lasts for more than a month, it can be considered chronic insomnia, which usually requires some sort action to remedy the situation.
- ▶ A fixation with sleep is a major problem for insomnia sufferers; for example, spending a lot of time trying to sleep, or feeling anxious about the consequences of not sleeping.
- ▶ People with insomnia will often fall into routines that make insomnia worse, such as watching TV in bed until the early hours, or having an irregular daytime schedule.
- ▶ Insomnia sufferers often underestimate the amount of sleep they get each night, further exacerbating their fixation on sleep.

As we can see, insomnia can be complex.

The different types of insomnia

Sometimes insomnia coexists with other conditions such as medical complaints or mental health problems. In such cases, using the recommendations in this book can bring about many benefits; for example, insomnia can make a person's subjective experience of anxiety worse. By using the exercises in this book, you may improve your sleep and therefore lessen your experience of anxiety.

As with all medical or psychological matters, it is important that you seek help from your GP if you feel any of the following factors might be implicated in your insomnia.

CHRONIC PAIN AND OTHER MEDICAL CONDITIONS

Chronic pain can lead to difficulties sleeping for obvious reasons. Where chronic pain is an issue, there is a specific self-hypnosis exercise that may help. Follow the relevant recommendations in Chapters 1–9 first, and then practise with the *self-hypnosis* exercise in Chapter 10. Self-hypnosis can be effective for pain relief, but you should discuss this with your GP first. Self-hypnosis should only be used in cases of chronic pain, never in cases of acute pain, or pain without an established medical diagnosis.

Insomnia that exists as a symptom or side-effect of another problem is known as *secondary* insomnia. An over-active thyroid or certain medications can cause problems with sleep, for example. In such cases, the recommendations outlined in this book may help. Although secondary insomnia exists as a result of something else, it can be addressed specifically, often with very good results.

DEPRESSION AND ANTIDEPRESSANTS

Depression can lead to insomnia: the most frequent complaint being early-morning wakening. Insomnia can make depression worse. The feelings of sadness, of emptiness, of feeling disengaged or uninterested in life grow stronger with sleeplessness. Insomnia can also interfere with antidepressant medications.

Following the exercises in this book can help in cases where insomnia coexists with depression. If you are receiving treatment for depression, many of the recommendations in this book may help. If you have any of the symptoms of depression, and you have not yet spoken to your doctor, it is strongly recommended that you do so. Symptoms of depression include:

▶ Frequent or consistent feelings of sadness, emptiness, upset or anger
▶ Withdrawing from the people you normally associate with
▶ Struggling with poor self-belief and motivation
▶ Self-neglect or struggles with personal hygiene
▶ Harmful thoughts about guilt, worthlessness or wanting the pain to stop
▶ No longer enjoying those things that used to give you pleasure
▶ Suicidal thoughts. (Note: if you have experienced any suicidal thoughts then consider contacting your GP immediately.)

Depression can be treated. You do not have to suffer indefinitely. Seeking assistance from your GP is the best place to start. If your insomnia is a depression-related problem, mention that to your GP and discuss the recommendations in this book. Your doctor is likely to recommend antidepressant medications. These medications vary in the effect they can have on insomnia: some worsen insomnia whereas others can improve a person's sleep. Again, the recommendations in this book may be able to help with that.

There are several exercises in this book that can help with anxiety. However, it is worth contacting your GP, or a mental health professional, if you have been experiencing excessive anxiety in day-to-day life. Anxiety can be generalized (worrying excessively about every little thing) or specific (for example, worrying about your health or social situations). If your experience of anxiety has persisted for more than six months, it may require some form of intervention.

The same advice stands if you are experiencing panic attacks regularly. Most people will experience some form of panic attack in their life. Regular panic attacks can cause insomnia, particularly if they occur while trying to sleep. Typical symptoms of panic attacks can include:

- ▶ Uncontrollable worry that lasts for a significant amount of time
- ▶ Palpitations, a rapidly beating heart or a pounding heart
- ▶ Sweating, trembling, shaking, feeling faint or dizzy
- ▶ Chest pains or nausea
- ▶ Feeling that everything is becoming detached, unreal or that you are not yourself
- ▶ Racing thoughts of panic and losing control
- ▶ Strong anxious feelings.

Sleeplessness can make a person's experience of anxiety worse. Anxiety experiences can make sleep difficult to achieve. It is recommended that you implement all of the recommendations in this book, paying particular attention to Chapter 6. However, if you have experienced any of the symptoms listed above for any length of time, contact your GP first.

In those cases where insomnia coexists with depression, or an anxiety or panic disorder, the exercises in this book will equip you with tools that can prevent a re-emergence of insomnia, should it clear up after a successful treatment. Insomnia does tend to come and go. The recommendations in this book can help in those instances.

Other sleep disorders

Insomnia is not the only sleep disorder that causes sleeplessness. Other sleep disorders include *sleep apnoea, restless leg syndrome* or *circadian rhythm sleep disorders*. These less common sleep disorders tend to be mistaken for insomnia. In fact, one criterion for the diagnosis of insomnia is an absence of other sleep disorders. Sleeplessness is a complex and multifaceted experience.

Some of the recommendations in this book can help with other sleep disorders; however, if you suspect you have a sleep disorder other than insomnia, then it is important that you contact your GP for further advice on treatment.

SLEEP APNOEA

Obstructive sleep apnoea is the most common breathing-related sleep disorder. Typical symptoms include loud snoring, frequent pauses in breathing lasting for 10 seconds or more, followed by a resumption in breathing. This resumption is often accompanied by loud gasps or violent movement. Usually obstructive sleep apnoea does lead to sleepiness during the day, but it is usually a person's partner who picks up on the symptoms; the sufferer is often unaware of their breathing difficulties.

If you or your partner suspect you have some of the symptoms described above, then it is important that you contact your GP for further advice and treatment.

RESTLESS LEG SYNDROME

Restless leg syndrome is characterized by an urge to move, usually with unpleasant sensations in the legs. It can feel painful, burning, or itchy, or as if insects are crawling over the skin. The cause is unknown, and some drugs such as antidepressants and antihistamines can make it worse. It is usually treated by neurologists or sleep specialists, and if you recognize any of the symptoms of restless leg syndrome, you should contact your GP for further advice or treatment.

CIRCADIAN RHYTHM SLEEP DISORDERS

Circadian rhythm sleep disorders are disturbances in the normal sleep–wake rhythm. The most frequent example of this is jet lag where, due to crossing time zones, our body clock no longer matches our new local time. This will result in sleeplessness, tiredness, fuzzy-headedness, mood changes, stomach upsets and the like. For the majority of people, travelling eastward is most difficult. The rate of adaptation, i.e. the time it takes to recover from jet lag, tends to be roughly one day per hour of time zone difference.

Some of the recommendations in this book can help with jet lag, particularly the *relaxation* exercises from Chapter 7.

Delayed sleep phase syndrome

Delayed sleep phase syndrome (DSPS) is a circadian rhythm sleep disorder, prevalent particularly in adolescents and young children. It is characterized by a difficulty in falling asleep before 2 a.m., and with a preferred waking time of around 10 a.m. People with delayed sleep phase syndrome will tend to suffer with sleep-onset insomnia and *hypersomnia*, which means feeling sleepy during the day. Remember, with insomnia, feeling excessively sleepy or actually falling asleep is uncommon. DSPS, where feeling sleepy and falling asleep can be common, causes a different set of daytime problems from insomnia.

The recommendations in this book can help with DSPS, but if your daytime symptoms typically include sleepiness, or actually falling asleep, you should contact your GP.

Advanced sleep phase syndrome

Advanced sleep phase syndrome (ASPS) is a rare circadian rhythm sleep disorder that affects roughly 1 per cent of middle-aged and older adults. It is characterized by habitually falling asleep some two to three hours earlier than desired, coupled with frequent waking during the night.

Treatment for this disorder involves exposure to bright light in the evening, delaying sleep. Some of the recommendations in this book can help. If you are experiencing ASPS, you should contact your GP for further advice and treatment.

Insomnia can exist on its own or in conjunction with physical or psychological conditions. It can be easy to spot or it can be wrongly diagnosed where in fact a different sleep disorder is present. In most cases, insomnia will lead to fatigue, rather than sleepiness, during the day. It is important to learn the difference between the two experiences and assess whether you have insomnia or a rarer sleep disorder; for example, delayed sleep phase syndrome.

Next, we shall take a look at a useful tool to help you overcome your sleeplessness: your *sleep diary.*

Keeping a sleep diary

A sleep diary is simply a record of your sleeping habits. You might think that you know precisely the amount of sleep you get each night. And yet, people who use sleep diaries invariably find the results surprising.

Do you check your bank statements? Some of us do. Many of us don't, perhaps afraid to track how much money is going out compared with how much is going in! The tracking of things can be unpopular. Perhaps, as humans, sometimes we prefer not to know.

The tracking of performance is incredibly useful. Consider the modern athlete. He or she will have every second of their performance, in training and competition, tracked and analysed. This allows their team of coaches to pinpoint strengths and weaknesses, areas for improvement and areas that are already at a peak performance.

Earlier in this chapter we mentioned sleep misperception. Sufferers of insomnia frequently underestimate the amount of sleep they get. If we are to overcome insomnia, we need more objective feedback. A sleep diary will allow us to know precisely what is going on. Just like the coach of a world-class athlete, we'll be able to pinpoint strengths and weaknesses, areas for improvement and areas that are already acceptable.

Using a sleep diary will fulfil two functions. It will allow us to get an objectively accurate overview of your insomnia. It is likely that you describe your insomnia in generalized terms, with statements such as, '*I only ever get five hours' sleep per night, maximum.*' Even in cases of chronic insomnia, the amount of sleep a person gets tends to vary from night to night. Keeping a sleep diary will allow you to challenge the negative, limiting thoughts you have about insomnia. After two weeks or so, any patterns inherent to your insomnia will begin to emerge. You will be able to see precisely where your sleep difficulties lie, and therefore you will be a step closer to addressing those problems.

Insight – using your sleep diary

Whenever I work with clients to help them overcome insomnia, I request that they start by using a sleep diary: it is far too useful a tool to ignore. Sometimes there will be some resistance on the client's part, which I can understand. For whatever reason, we can dislike starting new and unfamiliar things, especially when it involves filling in sheets of paper!

However, the sleep diary in this book is really simple and very easy to use. It will take just a couple of minutes, and over the coming weeks the information you record there will prove invaluable. We need a record of your sleeping habits if we are going to do our best work together.

Some people will look at this first recommendation and skip past it. *Does it really matter?* Yes! If you skip this bit, you will miss out later in this book. It is a simple task, and you will really benefit from it. I strongly recommend that you start using your sleep diary as soon as possible.

The second function your sleep diary will serve is to record your improvement. In the coming chapter(s), we are going to put in place changes that should dramatically improve your sleep. This improvement, change in other words, rarely follows a straight line:

▶ Sometimes, a person's recovery from a condition such as insomnia can be seen as a gentle, steady increase in the amount of sleep they get, consistently improving until they are fully recovered.

▶ More frequently, a person overcomes insomnia by phasing in and out of periods of good sleep, interspersed with periods of unsatisfactory sleep. As treatment progresses, the periods of good sleep last longer as the periods of unsatisfactory sleep decrease.

▶ Occasionally, a person's recovery might stall. They bumble along for a while without making any real progress. Then, something clicks into place and they make good progress from that point.

The reality is that our recovery from sleeplessness and insomnia often encompasses all of these forms of change. Keeping a simple, accurate and up-to-date sleep diary will help you track your progress. That will encourage you when things are going well, and remind you not to fall into bad habits if the amount of sleep you get worsens temporarily.

So, the advantages of keeping a sleep diary are:

▶ An accurate overview of how much sleep you are *actually* getting, dispelling any misperceptions you might have about your sleep pattern

- You will probably be surprised to learn that you get more sleep than it sometimes appears
- It will help you determine the problem areas that exist when it comes to your sleep
- It will track your recovery as you implement the changes in this book.

Are there any advantages to not keeping a sleep diary? I can think of only one.

- You will save yourself two to three minutes, each morning.

On balance, keeping a sleep diary would seem to make sense! Photocopy the table on the following page, making 12 copies. Keep those pages, plus something to write with, by the side of your bed within easy reach. Only accurate feedback is useful, so fill it out each morning. If you miss a day, don't guess, just skip that day and start again tomorrow.

Aim to make your answers as accurate as possible, but you don't need to sleep with a stop watch under your pillow! Give your best estimates the following morning, and they will be consistent enough.

The next tip is not strictly Neuro-linguistic Programming, but it will help. On a piece of paper or card, write the following in big letters and keep it with your sleep diary next to your bed:

GOOD MORNING! NOW PLEASE FILL IN YOUR SLEEP DIARY BEFORE YOU GET IN THE SHOWER!

In summary:

- Keep your sleep diary by the side of the bed, with a pen and perhaps something to rest on.
- Use a little note to remind you to fill it in each morning.
- Record information each morning as soon as possible after getting out of bed.
- If you forget to complete the diary on any given morning, leave that day blank and begin again tomorrow.
- Aim to fill it in each day for the next two to four weeks.

SLEEP DIARY

Day: _____ Date:_____

Please complete each morning when you wake up.

Sleep aids taken last night: x mg sleep aid / x units alcohol	3 units alcohol
Time I went to bed last night (if you got up again, list each time separately):	11.30 pm 12.50 am
Time it took to fall asleep (if you tried to several times, list each time separately):	20 min. 20 min.
Did I use the NLP exercises in Chapters 5–7 (as appropriate)?	
Number of times I awoke during the night (do not count your final waking):	2 times
Length of time spent trying to get back to sleep (list each arousal separately):	20 min. 12 min.
Did I use the NLP exercises in Chapters 5–7 (as appropriate)?	
Final waking time:	6.30 am
Time I got out of bed:	7.20 am
I woke up x minutes earlier / later than I wanted to (last waking):	30 min.
Quality of sleep on a scale of 1–5 (1 = very poor, 5 = excellent):	2

There is a blank version of this sleep diary provided on the following page so that you may photocopy it.

SLEEP DIARY

Day: _____ Date: _____

Please complete each morning when you wake up.

One sheet per day; fill out each morning.

Have a go

- ▶ Filling out your sleep diary is really simple; it will take less than 5 minutes every time.
- ▶ You'll see there is an example column, which makes it all self-explanatory.
- ▶ We'll go though each column now to make sure it all makes sense.

1 In the first row for that day: record any sleep aids, including alcohol before bed, that you took on the previous night (alcohol with an evening meal doesn't count as a sleep aid).

2 In the second row: record the time(s) you actually got into bed.

3 In the third row: estimate how long it took you to get to sleep.

4 In the fourth row: note whether you used any of the exercises in this book to help you fall asleep.

5 In the fifth row: note how many times (if any) that you woke. You do not need to count your final waking here, just times when you woke and then returned to sleep.

6 In the sixth row: note how long it took you to fall back to sleep after each period of waking.

7 In the seventh row: note whether you used any of the exercises in this book to go back to sleep.

8 In the eighth row: note your final waking time.

9 In the ninth row: record the time you actually got out of bed.

10 In the tenth row: make a note of the difference, in minutes, between your final waking time and your preferred waking time.

11 In the eleventh row: give an estimate of the quality of your sleep.

As you can see, it is very straightforward. Completing your sleep diary each day will make a tremendous difference to your efforts to overcome insomnia. If at any point you skip a day, re-read this chapter and regain your motivation. Filling in your sleep diary is a simple task, but it will form the framework for our subsequent work together.

In this first chapter we have learned about sleep: how it works and how it can sometimes go wrong. In the next chapter we will take a look at Neuro-linguistic Programming: what it is, where it came from and how it can help.

10 TIPS FOR SUCCESS

1 Insomnia is a major public health problem. This book has been designed to help you sleep better by offering simple recommendations that work.

2 Typically, sleep unfolds in 90-minute cycles, usually four or five cycles per night. Periods of deep, restorative, slow-wave sleep are followed by bursts of REM sleep. As the night progresses, the periods of deep slow-wave sleep get shorter, giving way to greater periods of REM sleep.

3 Sleep is driven by two independent but interacting processes: the circadian process and the homeostatic process.

4 The circadian process is driven by our body clock. It regulates the timing of sleep.

5 The homeostatic process builds pressure to sleep. This pressure increases with each hour that a person is awake, usually peaking around 16 hours after waking up in the morning. There is a correlation between the homeostatic process and the amount of restorative slow-wave sleep we get. It regulates the intensity of sleep.

6 Insomnia is the most common sleep disorder; it is characterized by difficulties falling asleep, difficulties staying asleep, or waking too early in the morning.

7 Insomnia is a combination of sleeplessness coupled with daytime frustration, anxiety, fatigue, impaired performance, and eventually exhaustion. It is uncommon to experience sleepiness during the day as a result of insomnia.

8 Insomnia can exist on its own, or in conjunction with a medical or psychological condition. If you suspect a medical or psychological condition is causing your insomnia, it is important to contact your GP for advice and treatment.

9 There are other sleep disorders that can often be confused with insomnia. Consult your GP if you recognize any of the other sleep disorder symptoms mentioned in this book.

10 Keeping a sleep diary will help you get a clearer and more objective view of your sleeplessness. It will help to track your recovery and assist with troubleshooting later. It is a tiny commitment which will really help in the long run.

HOW AM I GETTING ON?

▶ *Have you read and understood the information on sleep, the circadian process, and the homeostatic process? How does this information relate to your own difficulties with sleep?*

▶ *Have you checked to see whether, during the day, you feel sleepy or fatigued?*

▶ *Have you read and understood the information presented on insomnia: how it can be a stand-alone problem, or a problem in conjunction with other medical or psychological conditions?*

▶ *Have you read the information on other sleep disorders to check whether your problem is insomnia, or a different disorder?*

▶ *Have you photocopied the sleep diary, enough for two to four weeks, and placed it with a pen, and a reminder to fill it in, by your bed?*

By learning about sleep, how it works, and how it can go wrong, we have taken the first step towards beating insomnia with Neurolinguistic Programming. Using your sleep diary is the second step, and it is strongly recommended that you take it. It is easy, of course, to just read through a book such as this without implementing any of the recommendations. However, if you make a start now and follow the programme, you will have a much greater chance of success.

2

....

Exploring NLP

In this chapter you will learn:
- *the basics of NLP*
- *how NLP 'presuppositions' can change the way you think*
- *how models can help you better understand insomnia*
- *about NLP and learning.*

> *We don't see things as they are, but rather as we are.*
>
> Anaïs Nin

In the previous chapter we learned about sleep and sleeplessness: how sleep works and how it can go wrong. We then looked at reasons for using a sleep diary. It is a useful tool that will provide us with the feedback we need to overcome insomnia.

In this chapter we are going to learn about NLP. To begin, let's take a look at the basics: what it is, what it does, and how it can help.

What is NLP?

NLP stands for Neuro-linguistic Programming. It is a collection of mental techniques gathered together in order to bring about positive change:

- ▶ **Neuro** is a prefix used for topics relating to the brain, such as neuroscience, neurology, etc.
- ▶ **Linguistic** describes the study of human language.
- ▶ **Programming** is the provision of an ordered set of instructions or procedures.

Imagine a computer programmer working on a new software package. He would write a series of instructions, given to a computer in a particular sequence, in order for the software to work. This is known as programming.

Computer programs are written in different languages depending on the type of computer used. Our brains also run using language. Language can refer to the visual as well as the verbal: Egyptian hieroglyphics, for example. NLP can be described as *programming the brain using visual and spoken language*. Throughout this book you will be introduced to mental exercises, each designed to programme your brain for better sleep. With NLP, people quickly learn what it means to find real, positive change in their lives.

One of the great strengths of Neuro-linguistic Programming is the emphasis placed on visualization techniques. As we learn about these techniques together, the power of visualization will quickly become clear.

Insight – visualization

Have you ever watched Olympic athletes before their big race, going through their pre-race rituals? These rituals will include visualizing the race as they want it to unfold. As Usain Bolt put it, after setting a world record for the men's 100 metres, *'I just visualized and then executed my plan.'*

It makes sense that the athletes would be focusing on the race rather than, say, what they're going to have for dinner that night, or whether they've locked the back door! Also, it makes sense to focus on running the race well rather than badly. There will be a difference in performance levels between the athlete who confidently visualizes himself leaving the trailing pack behind, versus the athlete who anxiously worries about defeat. The first athlete is likely to prevail, whereas the second is likely to struggle.

Using visualization techniques to mentally rehearse performance will then improve that performance. NLP is very much focused on this fact.

And yet, there is more to NLP than exercises for reprogramming our brains. Neuro-linguistic Programming is also a collection of ideas: some original and some borrowed, underpinned by a philosophy of learning and understanding. Harnessing these ideas will help as you work through this book. They will inform your approach to making the changes you need.

For example, have you ever failed at anything? An exam? A driving test? We humans tend to hate and fear failure. Failure feels bad and we are often left blaming ourselves. We may find it difficult to motivate ourselves to try again. However, failure is a familiar experience to us all. Each time we try something new we run the risk of getting it wrong, certainly to begin with. Consider this 1921 quote from Thomas Edison, relating to his work on improving the lifespan of the electric light bulb:

After we had conducted thousands of experiments on a certain project without solving the problem, one of my associates, after we had conducted the crowning experiment and it had proved a failure, expressed discouragement and disgust over our having failed to find out anything. I cheerily assured him that we had learned something. For we had learned for a certainty that the thing couldn't be done that way, and that we would have to try some other way.

Famously persistent, Thomas Edison is stating that 'there is no failure, only feedback'. This is an idea often referred to in NLP. Let's consider it more closely for a moment.

What would happen if you looked at your insomnia in a different light? If, rather than becoming frustrated, instead, like Edison, you systematically tried different approaches to resolve it? An experiment. An opportunity to learn what works and what doesn't. Whether successful or otherwise, with each night you would learn from your experience and, at some point, you'd discover precisely what works for you. Instead, we tend to become anxious about our failures. Despondent. Certain that we are powerless to change things, and that our future efforts are also likely to fail.

Perhaps this fear of failure is something we acquire as we grow older. When first learning to tie our shoelaces, we persist until we get it right. There are many, many things that you learned to do as a child, simply by practising. Reading. Writing. Learning to speak. Learning to walk. As children, we move beyond the failures and frustrations of learning. As adults, we often forget to do this.

NLP 'presuppositions'

There is a lot of jargon in NLP. Even the name 'Neuro-linguistic Programming' can make a person's eyes glaze over! As we go through this book together, we'll demystify the jargon. The concepts of NLP aren't difficult to understand, even if some of the language seems unnecessarily complex at first.

There is no failure, only feedback is one of several ideas referred to in NLP. These ideas are known collectively as NLP presuppositions. A presupposition is simply an idea we suppose to be true. These ideas form a framework which, when harnessed, makes the *programming* part of NLP even more effective. Here are some examples of NLP presuppositions:

▶ *Having a choice is better than not having a choice.* This might seem obvious, but consider your insomnia for a moment. What could you do to give yourself the choice to fall asleep? This book is going to answer that question.

▶ *We have all of the resources we will ever need.* A resource is something you can draw on. At some stage in your life you have slept, and slept well. Your body inherently knows how to sleep, even if you feel you have lost that ability. This book is going to reconnect you with your ability to sleep soundly.

▶ *Your mind and body are parts of the same system.* Recently, medical science has started to recognize the connection between mind and body. It is now accepted that mental stress can inhibit the performance of the immune system, for example. Controlling your mind, something NLP is designed to do, is a major part of getting a good night's sleep.

There are several more such presuppositions that, together, form a philosophy for understanding, changing and improving our experience. As we go through our work together, these presuppositions will be woven through this book, always working towards helping you towards better sleep.

So, there are specific presuppositions woven through NLP. Guidelines, if you will. Collectively, these ideas contribute to, and reflect, a philosophy of learning and experimentation. To understand this, it helps to know where NLP came from, and how it evolved over the years.

Neuro-linguistic Programming was developed in the 1970s by a university lecturer, John Grinder, and an undergraduate student, Richard Bandler. It began as a study of some well-known psychotherapists of the day, in particular how they managed to achieve impressive results with their clients. From this study, Bandler and Grinder tried to describe the thoughts, feelings, language and behaviours of these therapists in order to teach other psychotherapists how to get similar results. As this work was expanded upon, NLP grew into a collection of practical ideas and techniques designed to be accessible to everybody, not just therapists.

In the 1980s, Bandler and Grinder acrimoniously ended their association, and lawsuits inevitably followed. By this point, a new generation of researchers and practitioners were exploring what NLP could do, continuing the tradition of experimental and practical research. Training schools were set up, and countless books written. Bandler and Grinder continued to work on Neuro-linguistic Programming separately. In the year 2000, they agreed to leave their professional differences behind them and each was recognized as 'the co-creator of NLP'.

From these obscure beginnings 30 years ago in California, NLP is now used in a wide range of fields, including sales and marketing, business communication, sports performance, psychotherapy and education. NLP is a collection of mental exercises, plus a broader framework of philosophical ideas, that arose from an attitude of curiosity, learning and practical experimentation. Just like Edison, as we work towards bringing an end to your insomnia, we will aim to find out what works for you, and what doesn't.

There is another area in NLP that will help you overcome insomnia: models.

Models in NLP

A model is a representation of something. Imagine an architect working on a new shopping centre. After the plans have been drawn, architectural models will be made. These miniature representations of the proposed building are used to understand better what it will finally look like. Clearly, the architectural model of the shopping centre isn't the actual shopping centre, instead it describes how the final building will look. Models help us improve our understanding of things by describing them.

Some models can be conceptual, wrought from the material of our understanding. A conceptual model's purpose is still to describe. Such models are useful tools to improve our understanding of matters, but they don't have to be completely accurate. The architectural model does not predict precisely how the final building will look. The same is true for conceptual models. However, models enrich our eventual understanding by giving us the opportunity to look at things in a different way.

Let's take a look at one such model now, and all will become clear. The Neurological Levels Model, developed in 1990 by researcher Robert Dilts, can help shed some light on your insomnia by helping you look at it in a different way.

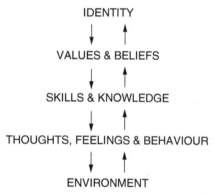

IDENTITY

VALUES & BELIEFS

SKILLS & KNOWLEDGE

THOUGHTS, FEELINGS & BEHAVIOUR

ENVIRONMENT

In this modified version of Dilts' Neurological Levels Model, each level has an impact on the levels above and the level(s) below. Let's run insomnia through this model, and see what we get. We'll begin with environment, and work our way up the levels. (We could have an interesting discussion about the various criticisms of this model, but let's save that for another time; it is a useful tool to describe, and therefore understand, things more thoroughly.)

ENVIRONMENT

How does our environment affect sleep? An obvious example would be trying to sleep in a noisy or uncomfortable place. Many people find it difficult to sleep on a plane, for instance. People often find it difficult to sleep when it is too hot, or too cold. Where insomnia is concerned, keeping your environment cool, quiet and dark can really make a difference.

THOUGHTS, FEELINGS AND BEHAVIOUR

According to the model we're using, changing our environment will have an effect on our thoughts, feelings and behaviour. This is borne out in real life: making your sleeping environment more comfortable is likely to affect the behaviour of falling asleep. The reverse is also true. Changing your behaviour will affect your environment, and we will look at this in more detail later.

What other behaviours are tied in to insomnia? Some are subtle, some not. If tomorrow you drank 15 cups of strong coffee, would this make it more likely, or less likely, that you'd sleep easily? There are many behaviours that affect sleep: good habits that will definitely help and bad habits that it would help to eliminate.

SKILLS AND KNOWLEDGE

Our behaviours are, at least in part, governed by our skills and knowledge. Most people agree that learning to relax can help with insomnia. If you increase your ability to relax at bedtime, you're more likely to fall asleep.

The exercises in this book will take some practice. By repeatedly using the exercises in this book (practice), you'll become skilful at them. Acquiring new skills and knowledge relating to sleep is going to increase the likelihood of sleep.

BELIEFS AND VALUES

A belief is simply an idea that we hold as being true. We have many beliefs: some vital and some obscure, some rational and some contradictory. Beliefs have a profound effect on our relationship with the world. Our self-image, our perception of our strengths and weaknesses, what we're worth, our chances in life and our place in the world will be affected by what we believe. It is our beliefs that define what we expect from life and ourselves.

Beliefs aren't real; they are just ideas. Many, many years ago, it was believed that the Earth was flat. We can feel amused by this inaccurate belief now and yet, you will certainly carry a whole raft of inaccurate beliefs of your own. Your beliefs, inaccurate and otherwise, govern your thoughts, feelings and behaviours in subtle ways.

Our beliefs inform our view of the future, in terms of probabilities and even inevitabilities. As somebody who has struggled with insomnia, you may have gone to bed feeling certain that a night of tossing and turning awaited you. As a result of believing that, the likelihood of it happening increases: a self-fulfilling prophecy. Your beliefs about sleep and sleeplessness are at the heart of your insomnia, and much of this book will be focused on changing them for the better.

A value is a special kind of belief: an indication of what is important to us. Some people value money. Some people value security. Some people value love. There are as many different values as there are people. As Richard Bandler (the co-creator of NLP) once put it, *'Values are what get us out of bed in the morning.'*

Do you value sleep? Instinctively you may wish to answer yes. If so, are you ready to take the required steps to make sleep easier? Some of the recommendations in this book might feel like a wrench at first. Sometimes, we need to remember what we value: to live in concert with our values is to live a happier life.

IDENTITY

Taken together, our environment, our behaviours, our skills and knowledge, our values and our beliefs all contribute to our sense of identity, our sense of who we are. If a person identifies themselves as *an insomniac*, then this sense of identity will affect their beliefs and values about sleep, their ability to sleep, their behaviours connected with sleep, and even how they organize the environment in which they sleep. How we see ourselves impacts massively on what happens in our lives.

So consider this: do you see yourself as somebody who cannot sleep easily? If so, it is likely that this *top-level* identification is creating problems on each of the levels we have identified. The aim of our work together, ultimately, is for you to see yourself as somebody who sleeps easily, naturally, consistently and confidently.

Insight – the Neurological Levels Model

Throughout this book we'll be aiming to optimize your environment; your thoughts, feelings and behaviours; your skills and knowledge; your values and beliefs; and even your identity for better sleep. By being this thorough we are doing everything we can to guarantee your eventual success.

Ultimately, the Neurological Levels Model *is* just a model. There are valid criticisms, but it serves to organize the knowledge and exercises presented in this book in a meaningful way.

Have a go

Insomnia is not just sleeplessness. It can be a complex experience, with many contributing factors. To help you understand this, go through the various levels of the Neurological Levels Model once more, with a pen and paper to hand, and write down any factors you think may be contributing to your insomnia. It could be problems with your sleeping environment, certain bad habits (behaviours), an inability to relax, limiting beliefs or values relating to sleep, or even identifying yourself as a 'hopeless insomniac'. Take a bit of time and see if you can spot where some of your difficulties with sleep stem from.

NLP and learning

Learning is a natural thing to do. There are many things you have learned so far in your life. And many more things to come. It would be impossible for you not to learn lessons in life. So what does learning mean?

We can state what learning isn't. For a start, learning is not the same as being taught. Being taught, by a teacher at school, for example, may or may not result in learning. It depends on the skill of the teacher and the involvement of the pupil. Where there is a mismatch between these elements, the pupil will be frustrated, anxious or bored. Few of us are good at learning simply by having things explained to us.

With that in mind, is simply reading this book likely to result in your learning how to overcome your insomnia? Reading through this book and then leaving it on a bookshelf somewhere is unlikely to help. We learn best by *actively* acquiring small chunks of knowledge and then applying them. The temptation might be to read this book, several chapters at a time, without really *acting* on it. Without even taking it in. Instead, try to read just one chapter at a time, and complete the exercises in each chapter. When taken a step at a time, learning is much more likely to happen.

According to NLP, there are four stages we go through when learning. In our efforts to help you overcome your insomnia, you'll be asked to try new things. Learning can take time. To understand this, let's imagine that we are learning to drive for the first time.

UNCONSCIOUS INCOMPETENCE

The beginning of the learning experience. In our example of learning to drive, this initial stage reflects a complete lack of competence at driving, and a lack of awareness as to what driving entails. Think back to the very first time you sat behind the wheel of a car: not knowing what the various controls do, what the pedals are for; not even knowing how to start the car. A complete lack of competence and a complete lack of awareness.

CONSCIOUS INCOMPETENCE

The second stage of learning. With some practice, we have gained an awareness of what we're trying to learn: how to drive the car. We now at least have some idea of what driving is about. That isn't to say we are particularly good at it. Mistakes are made. We're still causing occasional panic to our driving instructor! Still incompetent in fact. And yet, measurable improvement comes quickly at this stage; it is much more difficult for an expert to improve, compared with the quick gains made by a novice.

CONSCIOUS COMPETENCE

Here, we're getting pretty good at driving. We still have to think about it. We need to concentrate, and our efforts aren't always consistent. However, this stage of learning is satisfying. Our efforts are starting to pay off and we know what we're doing. Parts of driving now become automatic, in that we don't need to think about changing gear, or checking the mirrors, it just ... happens.

UNCONSCIOUS COMPETENCE

With practice, reading, learning and understanding, we've arrived at a point where our knowledge is well bedded in. We can drive well and even do other things at the same time, such as holding a conversation with fellow passengers, or listening to music. Driving happens naturally, smoothly, and our ability is far in advance of when we first started. Our high level of competence means we can drive well without being fully conscious of what we are doing. Our unconscious is doing it for us.

* * *

Things aren't just going to change in an instant; learning is a process that we have to go through. Throughout this book you will be introduced to new ways of doing things: exercises, techniques, ideas, all of which should help you overcome your problems with insomnia. Allow yourself the time to take this information in, and experiment with it. Learn what works, what doesn't. By giving yourself the time and space to learn what works for you, you're giving yourself the best chance of reaching an *unconscious competence* with the exercises in this book. Arriving at that stage will mean much better sleep.

•••

Insight – engaging with the exercises

You can't learn to drive a car by reading about driving. The journey from unconscious incompetence to unconscious competence requires interaction, experimentation and consideration. You will become competent with the techniques in this book quickly, providing you give them a try.

Some of the people who read this book will not engage with the exercises in any meaningful way. Instead of trying to learn, they will just passively read, eventually putting the book to one side. The result? Sleeplessness will persist and an opportunity to change will have been missed. Don't be one of those people. Complete what you have begun.

•••

Ultimately, you just need to be patient and open-minded. Try the techniques and exercises you find in these pages, and be willing to practise and experiment. With a little persistence, it will all make sense. Some exercises will work very well, in fact. When something works well for you, take some time to understand how it works. Similarly, if something doesn't work so well, consider what you could have tried differently, or move on to something else.

So, in this chapter we have explored the basics of Neuro-linguistic Programming. In the next chapter, we will look at what NLP *does* and how we can get it working for you.

10 TIPS FOR SUCCESS

1 NLP stands for Neuro-linguistic Programming. It is a collection of ideas and mental techniques, gathered together in order to bring about positive change.

2 Visualization is used by many elite athletes to improve their performance. Many NLP techniques employ visualization as well.

3 NLP presuppositions are useful guidelines for living a more effective life. For example, approaching your insomnia with the view that *there is no failure, only feedback,* would enable you to find out systematically what helps you to sleep better.

4 There is no failure, only feedback! Remember this presupposition as you experiment with the recommendations in this book. If things don't work straight away, look to learn from the experience. What could you do differently?

5 We can use models to help us understand how things work, particularly in relation to insomnia, its causes and its solutions.

6 We can organize human experience into a system of levels that affect and interact with one another: our environment, our behaviours, our skills and capabilities, our values and beliefs, and our identity.

7 Looking at insomnia in this way enables us to thoroughly understand the various issues that might be in play.

8 Learning is not the same as being taught. In order to learn effectively, it is best to be active rather than passive, and to take things a step at a time. So, rather than ploughing on to the next chapter, why not go through this chapter again, with a pen and paper to hand, in order to pick out the bits that seem most useful to you?

9 You will encounter many exercises in the coming pages. The best advice possible is to actually do them!

10 The sad truth is, some people will give up before completing this book. Some will skip past the exercises. Don't be one of them. Finish what you have started, and your chances of success are as high as they could be. You *can* get to sleep at night. All you need to do is make a start.

HOW AM I GETTING ON?

▶ *Have you reviewed your attempts to sleep with* there is no failure, only feedback *in mind? When you look at what you've tried in the past, what can you learn? What could you do differently?*

▶ *When you look at your insomnia using the Neurological Levels Model, what becomes clear? Are you able to identify where some of the problems lie; for example, your sleeping environment, or your beliefs about sleep?*

▶ *Have you fully resolved to do the exercises in this book? Many people will not. Their chances of overcoming insomnia will reflect that choice. You can choose to be different. You can choose to succeed and sleep more easily.*

Without action, how can there be real learning? With that in mind, unless you can answer yes to the three questions above, the best advice possible is to read the chapter again and do the exercises. If you complete the exercises in this book, your sleeping can improve.

3

···

Making NLP work for you

In this chapter you will learn:
- *about the different ways in which NLP can help you sleep*
- *how to use submodalities – the building blocks of your thoughts*
- *how to change your feelings*
- *how to program me your mind to fill in your sleep diary.*

   NLP is whatever works.

Robert Dilts

Understanding what something is and knowing how to use it are two different things. You may know what the Large Hadron Collider is but unless you are a gifted physics professor, it's unlikely that you'd know how to use one! Sometimes NLP can sound really complicated. In reality, it is very easy to put into practice. The only tool you need is your mind.

How NLP can help you sleep

Neuro-linguistic Programming rarely focuses on why you do things. Instead it focuses on *how* you do things. How do you find it difficult to sleep? How do you find it easier to sleep? By answering these questions we can focus on solutions, not problems. Your insomnia is not a random experience and the solution to it will reflect that.

As we go through our work together, you will be presented with exercises designed to gently change the way you think, the way you feel and the way you behave. As a result, it will be easier to put in place the solutions to your insomnia. What are these solutions? Some you will recognize; some will be new to you.

SLEEP EDUCATION

In Chapter 1 we discussed sleep, and sleeplessness, thoroughly. By learning about sleep, myths will be dispelled and your understanding of insomnia will be more nuanced, more realistic. Sleep education means having a clear, rational understanding of what sleep is and what it means to get enough of it. Using your sleep diary will also help with this.

Insomnia can be complex and personal. A sound sleep education will help you overcome any misconceptions you might have; barriers can be broken down and better sleep can be achieved. NLP is incredibly useful for making these types of changes. Much of NLP focuses on how we think about things. There will be specific exercises to practise.

SLEEP HYGIENE

Sleep hygiene is the name given to a collection of recommendations that focus on your sleeping environment and those habits which affect sleep, such as sticking to a regular rising time. You have probably encountered sleep hygiene recommendations before. In this book, you will be presented with a thorough list of improvements to make, and the tools required to make them.

Knowing what to do and actually doing it are two different things. Neuro-linguistic Programming will help because making such changes can feel daunting, and we often lack the motivation to act. Using some simple NLP techniques, you'll feel ready to act on the recommendations in this book at your own pace.

CHANGING YOUR STATE

Anxious thoughts and feelings are common causes of insomnia. We will explore techniques designed to overcome short-term and long-term anxiety. People with insomnia often acquire an irrational fear of sleeplessness. The exercises in Chapter 6 will help. We will then look to quieten your mind when you have certain worries in life, including worries about the consequences of insomnia.

Much of NLP is focused on state-control: learning how to think and feel differently. If you can gain control of your thoughts and feelings, you can gain control of your actions and therefore your life. This book will teach you about other resourceful states. How to get into a motivated state, how to get into a drowsy state and even how to get into a hypnotic state.

RELAXATION

There is a difference between feeling tired and feeling sleepy. The difference is relaxation. In Chapter 7 you will be presented with a list of techniques designed to help you feel drowsy, relaxed and ready to sleep. You will also learn about the beneficial effects of guided imagery.

Self-hypnosis has been shown to have a beneficial effect on a person's well-being. We will explore this in more detail later. In Chapter 10 we will practise a highly effective self-hypnosis technique designed to help you sleep more easily. If you suffer from chronic pain, this exercise will be of particular benefit.

TRANSFORMING NEGATIVE BELIEFS

We often underestimate the profound effect our beliefs have on our life. You will have certain beliefs about your insomnia which are contributing to the difficulties you are experiencing. In Chapter 8 we will look at the nature of belief and how it limits us. Change your beliefs and everything else will follow.

GOOD SLEEP HABITS FOR CHILDREN

Helping your children sleep better is only going to help you sleep better! If your children struggle to sleep, we'll look at what can be done to help. Children can be taught to sleep more easily.

* * *

Which of these different solutions might be particularly helpful for you? Over the coming chapters, we will work together to implement a thorough programme for change. Neuro-linguistic Programming will make these changes seem straightforward.

We mentioned earlier that NLP focuses on how you do things. To begin to understand how NLP can help, let's look at this in more detail.

Consider a typical insomnia sufferer. A busy job. A relationship with her boss that involves a lot of pressure. Too much work to complete, not enough time and no real control over her workload. With a young family to provide for, money is tight and she has little time to relax. These typical stresses and strains take their toll. Her diet consists of sugary or starchy foods, and endless cups of coffee.

Exercise? Just the walk each morning from her front door to her car. A car that is becoming more and more expensive to run. Not to mention that the insurance renewal is due next month. It's no wonder she can't sleep!

We could ask this unfortunate lady, '*Why can't you sleep?*' Perhaps she could identify some, or even all, of the factors mentioned above. Identifying the various factors behind a person's insomnia is useful, but only up to a point. We could advise her to change her job, her lifestyle, her car. In reality, however, such advice isn't particularly practical. 'Why' hasn't got us very far.

Let's ask this person '*How* do you struggle to sleep?' With some consideration, she will be able to describe precisely what thoughts, feelings and behaviours lead up to her sleepless nights. She'll be able to describe precisely how she worries about her workload, and the feelings of anxiety these thoughts create. She'll be able to describe the cravings she experiences before she has her next cup of coffee. The frustration at being unable to relax, and so on. By asking her *how*, rather than *why*, we get a much richer understanding of the problem, which means we can address those things that are under her control. She cannot control her boss, but she can control how she thinks about her boss. This is what NLP is all about.

Put simply, answers to questions beginning with *why* can give us the cause and effect relationship between one thing and another, and that can be useful. Answers to questions beginning with *how* can give us the solution, and that is invaluable. Neuro-linguistic Programming focuses on solutions. How do you get motivated? How do you believe in your ability to sleep? How do you relax? How do you overcome difficulties in your life?

OVERCOMING DIFFICULTIES IN YOUR LIFE

Have a go
Think about something you have overcome in your life. Something difficult. Something you are glad is over and which taught you to be stronger as a result. Ask yourself the following questions:

► How did I overcome that?
► How did I *do something beneficial?*

Ask yourself *how* repeatedly. How did I make this happen? How did that change? As you ask these questions, pay particular attention to the word *just*. There is no just, in reality. The word *just* is an indicator that there is more going on beneath the surface. Here is an example:

An example of a difficult time:	*Getting over a relationship break-up.*
How did I overcome that?	*In time, it became easier and I just moved on.*
How did it become easier?	*It hurt less. I didn't think about it as much.*
How did it hurt less?	*I started thinking about other things.*
How did I start thinking about other things?	*I focused on what was good in my life: family, friends...*
How did I focus on	*I decided to put him out of my mind, and when he*
what was good in my life?	*popped into my head, I told him to go away! Then I would think about something nice instead.*

We can see in this example that the person in question was able to replace negative, hurtful thoughts about her ex-boyfriend with nicer thoughts to do with her friends and family. This is a skill she has. If she were struggling with insomnia, she could apply the same process. Instead of focusing on the insomnia, and how bad it felt, she could replace those thoughts with something that felt nicer, such as the fact that she could have a nice, relaxing bath when she got home. It's the same process, albeit in a different context, and it would be one of the tools that would work well for her.

Take some time now to think about a past adversity you have overcome, and use the questioning technique above to determine *how* you managed it. From there, consider how you can use that experience to help with this programme.

Making NLP work for you

The strength of NLP lies in its flexibility. For this book to be effective, we need to get these techniques working for you. NLP is adaptable; it is most effective when tailored to your way of thinking. With NLP, there is no right way (or wrong way)... just your way.

Insight – make these exercises your own

Some of the exercises in this book will make an incredible difference, whereas others might seem less effective. We are unique individuals with our own thoughts, feelings and behaviours. Our aim with these techniques is to make them your own. A *one size fits all* approach would be much less effective. All you need is a little practice, a little imagination and a little experimentation.

It's like when you first learned to write: it takes a bit of concentration at first, but we each find our own style of handwriting. Learning happens naturally.

In order to make this book work for you, in order to overcome your sleeplessness and get a good night's rest, you need to follow a golden rule:

Actually do the exercises!

It is tempting to skip past the exercises, thinking, 'I'll try them later'. Instead, read this book, ideally with a pen and paper to hand, with an attitude of wanting to get involved. Wanting to practise and try it out for yourself. You can learn to overcome insomnia. The best advice is to read actively, not passively. There is nothing to lose and lots to gain.

People learn best by doing. Play around with the steps and ideas in each exercise until you get the right feeling and the sense that it's working. Insomnia is all about feeling (feeling too awake, feeling too anxious, not feeling sleepy enough) and so are the techniques you'll read about. Practise. Experiment. Try out each exercise, at least several times, until it either gels with your way of thinking, or until you feel certain that a different exercise will work better. Remember: you'll get back what you put in. Give each technique a chance to work for you.

Submodalities – the building blocks of your thoughts

Our minds are always generating thoughts. We might not always be aware of those thoughts; in fact, often we are not. Thoughts run through our mind regardless. If we can say anything about our minds, it is that they generate thoughts prodigiously.

What do you think about the most? Again, the scope is endless and people will experience many thoughts, good and bad, comforting and scary, positive and negative, aspirational and limiting. And, of course, all of the points in between. We think all of the time about all kinds of things. This is what it is to be human, in a sense.

What we think, and how we think it, has a massive impact on our lives. Our thoughts can be clear, bright, insistent. Sometimes they can be calm, dim, diffuse. NLP can help by changing the structure of our thoughts, which then changes our experience, including our experience of insomnia. So, let's look at *how* you think about things.

As you know, we have our five senses: sight, hearing, touch, smell and taste. We use these senses to, well, sense the outside world. We also use these senses internally: when thinking, day dreaming, working things out, remembering, fantasizing and so on. In NLP terms, these sensory thoughts are called *modalities*.

Let's try an exercise.

PRACTISING WITH SUBMODALITIES (PART ONE)

Have a go
In a moment, I'll ask you to close your eyes and think about being on a beach. Take a good 10 seconds at least, relax into it and really involve yourself in the *detail* of being on a beach. Make it a nice daydream; you can use memories of being on a beach to help get into it. Close your eyes and try the exercise now.

***

What was the first *detail* that you thought of? Was it an image, a sound or a feeling? Perhaps:

▶ The brightness of the sky? The colour of the sea?
▶ The sound of seagulls? Perhaps the sound of waves lapping against the beach?
▶ The warmth of the sun against your skin? The feeling of relaxing on holiday?

- The smell of the ocean?
- The taste of eating a delicious ice-cream while sitting on the beach?

Second, what was the most vivid aspect of the experience? What stood out the most? Was it what you saw, heard, or felt? If you're reading with a pen and paper to hand (well done!), set out your page in two columns, as shown below, and record your answers, noting the senses used.

First thing(s) noticed   Most vivid aspect(s)

_____   _____

_____   _____

_____   _____

_____   _____

Here we've established the first sense you used (the first thing thought about) and your preferred sense (the most vivid aspect).

Jargon buster – submodalities

Modality just means a *mode of thinking*: pictures, sounds, feelings, smells and tastes. It is with these modalities that you experience your thoughts and feelings in your mind.

Submodalities are the qualities your thoughts possess. Later, we'll be exploring these qualities, such as the brightness of any pictures, the volume of any sounds and the strength of any feelings. So:

- *Modality* means a thought that uses a specific sense, e.g. picturing a loved one (sense used: sight).
- *Submodalities* are specific qualities about that sensory thought, e.g. picturing your loved one brightly and in colour.

Don't worry too much about the jargon. NLP is really easy to do. So, people think with their senses. Not always, but often enough for it to be important, particularly when it comes to insomnia. Let's look at sensory thoughts again. This time we're going to identify and alter the qualities, the submodalities, of your thoughts.

Have a go

In a moment, close your eyes and think about something important to you: your children, your work, an enjoyable hobby perhaps. You get the idea. Again, relax into it and think about the detail. Make it a pleasant daydream. Take a good 10 seconds or so and try to involve all of your senses: seeing, hearing and feeling as best as you can. Let's try that now.

***

So, how did you think about your chosen topic? What did you see, hear and feel? On a piece of paper, set out two columns as shown below. Use the first column to note your answers.

Picture: _____ Qualities: _____

Sounds:_____ Qualities: _____

Feelings: _____ Qualities: _____

Don't worry if you struggled with a particular sense, such as making clear pictures or hearing sounds. With these exercises there is no right or wrong; we are all individuals with different styles, abilities and preferences. The point is to think about it vividly. However you think is right for you.

If there were pictures, what did you notice about them? Were they bright or dim? Moving or still? Did you see yourself in the picture (otherwise known as *dissociated*) or were you looking at the scene through your own eyes as if you were there (otherwise known as *associated*)?

What about the quality of any sounds you heard: loud or quiet? Close by or distant?

Finally, what feelings did you feel, if any? Where were those feelings in your body? Your stomach or your chest perhaps? Were they strong or weak? Heavy or light?

Now use the second column on your paper to note the qualities of your thoughts. If you need to, feel free to close your eyes and run through the exercise again. It's all good practice!

***

Excellent. Now, we're going to go through this scene again. This time, however, try the following:

▶ If there are pictures, try making them brighter, and then dimmer. More colourful, and then less colourful. If the pictures are moving, make them stop, and vice versa.

▶ Taking any sounds, make them louder and then quieter; closer to you and then further away.

▶ Finally, notice any feelings, and see if you can make them stronger, or weaker.

At this stage we're just experimenting. By changing the qualities of our sensory thoughts, we're practising using the most important tool we have: our mind. So, spend a little time picturing the scene again, relaxing into it, and work out which submodalities you can change, and what effect changing them has.

＊

What did you manage to change? Did you try to make pictures brighter or more colourful? Did you try to alter the sounds and feelings? Some people find that making these simple changes massively alters their experience of the daydream, whereas others report little difference. Later in this book we'll work out precisely which of your thoughts we need to change in order to have the most impact on your insomnia.

When it comes to your thinking, it doesn't matter if you make clear pictures, or if you only hear your own voice chattering away. It doesn't matter if you feel strong feelings, or feel no feelings at all. What is important is how these things affect your experience of being you. NLP works best when it is tailored to your way of doing things; changing *how* you think can really make a difference.

SPINNING FEELINGS (PART ONE)

We often refer to our feelings using language that describes movement: a sinking feeling, a rising anger. We speak of a throbbing headache or a shooting pain. Of fuzzy or tingling sensations. Feelings *move* through our body. We might not always be aware of the movement, but typically they do. If a person has a tight knot of tension in their stomach, they might feel that it just sits there. Tight knots also move, even if the movement is difficult to discern. It could be that the knot *rotates*, moving forwards, backwards, clockwise or anti-clockwise. If you don't find it easy to describe your feelings in terms of movement, it can help to use your hands to gesture how the feeling might be moving through your body.

Have a go

In a moment we are going to revisit the exercise above, where you thought, in vivid detail, about something important to you. This time spend up to a minute or so really getting into it. Allow yourself to relax a little, make the pictures as bright and bold as you can, and make it so you're associated into the picture, so it feels like you are there. If there are sounds, make them as clear as you can. Remember, this is all good practice for the exercises we'll be using later in this book.

When you're really into the visualization, notice the feelings going on in your body. Pay particular attention to your stomach, your chest, the back of your legs, your arms and hands, the front and back of your neck, and your face. Note especially the pathway that the feelings seem to move along. For example, this could be a feeling which rises through your torso or a feeling that spins tightly in your stomach or chest. Pay attention to how the feelings seem to move.

Try to discern the various qualities, the submodalities, of the feelings you notice, and record your answers below. It could be that the feelings you have during this exercise do not seem to have certain qualities. For example, the feeling might not have a particular heat to it (or it might feel very hot or cold). As before, there are no right or wrong answers. This is about learning. Let's try it now. Take a moment to close your eyes, relax and revisit the visualization where you thought vividly about something important to you.

***

Note your answers to the questions below on your sheet of paper:

Where was the feeling strongest? _____
(e.g. stomach, chest, etc.)

What type of feeling was it?_____
(happiness, fear, excitement, etc.)

What texture did it have?_____
(tingly, spiky, smooth, etc.)

What temperature did it have? _____
(hot, cold, no temperature, etc.)

Was it a wide feeling or narrow?_____

Was it fast moving or slow?_____

How did the feeling move? _____
(upwards, downwards, clockwise, anti-clockwise)

How intense was the feeling?_____
(use a scale of 1–10)

Any physiological changes?_____
(breathing, pulse, body temperature, etc.)

If the feeling had a colour, what would it be? _____
(e.g. red, blue, green, no colour?)

Did you manage to spend a minute or so on the exercise? What we're achieving here is a deeper understanding of the feelings that you have. Feelings are key to sleeplessness: anxiety, frustration, feeling too alert, not feeling drowsy enough. By connecting with your feelings, you can begin to control them. We can then start to build feelings that will aid sleep.

SPINNING FEELINGS (PART TWO)

Have a go

We are going to try this exercise one final time. Again you'll be asked to think vividly about something important to you. You can choose the same topic as before, or you can work with something new. Spend a minute or so really getting into it. Make the pictures bright and colourful, and try to associate yourself fully in the scene, so it feels like you're there, looking out through your own eyes.

This time, we're going to work with the feelings in order to decrease or increase the sensations. To do this, imagine lying in a bath. You could reach into the bath, scoop up handfuls of water and create waves. In this exercise, when you start to feel bodily feelings, note how they move (clockwise, anti-clockwise, up, down, or whichever) and then, using your mind to reach into the feeling, move it around faster, just as if you were making waves in water. Imagine making the width of the feeling wider. If there is a colour, imagine making it more vivid, more intense. Take a few moments to get your head around this. With a little perseverance you'll be changing feelings in no time.

Then, try the opposite. Attempt to move the feelings backwards, so they move against themselves. See if you can make the feelings narrower and, if there is a colour, less intense.

Let's try that now, and we'll see where it takes us.

***

How did you get on? It probably took you a little while to get into it. With a bit of practice, you will be able to change your feelings at will. If you can control your feelings, then you are much better placed to find sleep more easily.

How submodalities will help you sleep

Everything starts with a thought. The words you are reading. The book those words are printed in. The chair or settee on which you're sitting. The computer on which this book was written. Our experience of being alive is an experience we have with our minds. Our minds are full of preconceptions, particularly relating to the obstacles we will face in life. You will have preconceptions relating to your chances of getting a good night's sleep tonight. However, this future event, this future sleeplessness, does not yet exist. This future only exists in your mind.

But you might think, 'Hang on! I know I'll struggle to sleep tonight.' This knowledge of the future, a thing which only exists in your mind, is a generalization based on your past experiences, experiences which now also only exist in your mind. This statement isn't designed to denigrate, belittle or disbelieve your experiences. Far from it. To suffer with chronic and debilitating insomnia robs us of our vitality, of our quality of life. There is no criticism intended when pointing out the mental component to your insomnia. Instead, we can recognize that the solution to your sleeplessness will also come from your mind.

By using the submodality exercises we're learning about now, we'll be able to change the way you think and feel about sleep. From hopeless to hopeful. From anxious to relaxed. From beliefs that are limiting and self-perpetuating, to beliefs that are far more rational. To free your mind of misconceptions and limitations is a huge part of the battle.

Sleep is a natural thing for us to do. It does not exist outside of us, it is something that our body knows how to do. Alongside breathing or the regular beat of your heart, sleeping is one of the most natural things you do. You can be reconnected with that innate ability. Changing how you think will play a major part in that.

Insight – people do change

Over the years, in my capacity as a therapist, I've seen many people learn to sleep more easily; often people with terrible, chronic insomnia. You might have certain beliefs about your sleeplessness that hold you back, but insomnia can be beaten. This change might be surprisingly quick and simple, or you might need to give yourself time. Either way, remember that people change all the time, which means you can change, too. Keep an open mind, and let's see what we can learn together.

Let's take some of the elements we have discussed in this chapter and put them together. We learned that NLP is concerned with how we do things. We saw that changing the submodalities of our thoughts changes our experience at that time. Therefore, by using submodality exercises to change your thinking, specifically focusing on how to sleep well, you will ultimately be free of insomnia.

We can all do something well. It doesn't have to be earth-shattering or ground-breaking; it could be something relatively simple, mundane even. The point is, there is something that you can do well, and you know that you can do it well. It could relate to your work or a hobby. It could relate to being a parent or a good friend. Take a moment and think of something that you know you can do well. Choose something that you can imagine doing. When you have come up with an answer, write it on your piece of paper under the heading 'This is something I know I can do well'. Again, it doesn't need to be particularly exciting, it just needs to be something you are convinced you can do well.

Ideally, you've chosen something you can imagine doing. If not, have another think. Typical answers could include things such as driving, decorating, being a good friend or playing sport.

In a moment's time we are going to elicit the submodalities of your conviction: the way you imagine something you are convinced you can do. Take your time, and repeat the exercise a few times. There is no rush. Just as in the earlier exercises, relax, get into it and really let yourself connect with your imagination.

Have a go

In this exercise, notice the images, sounds and sensations that you experience as you think about your chosen topic. When you've spent some time immersed in the visualization, go through the list of submodalities below and note down your observations on a sheet of paper. You may want to use a pencil for this, as these answers may change as your visualization skills improve. Repeat this exercise a few times, get into it and be as thorough as you can be. First, pay attention to the quality of the image(s).

Number of images?_____
(one image, several images, etc.)

Moving or still?_____
(clear movement, kind of moving, totally still, etc.)

Fast movement or slow?_____

Colour or black-and-white? _____
(full vivid colour, washed out, sepia, black-and-white, etc.)

Bright images or dim?_____

Focused images or fuzzy? _____
(very focused, more focused in the middle, very fuzzy, etc.)

Size of the images?_____
(life-size, TV screen-size, somewhere in between the two?)

Location in your mind's eye?_____
(directly in front, panoramic, off to the left or right, above or below the eye-line?)

Close images or far away?_____
(did the images seem right in front of you, or in the distance?)

Was there a border?_____
(a coloured border around the image, no border, fuzzy around the edges, etc.)

3D images or flat?_____
(like real life, as on a TV screen, somewhere in between the two?)

Shape of the images?_____
(square, rectangular, oval, etc.)

How did you get on? Remember, people make all types of mental image, from very clear, crisp, full-colour images, to fuzzy black-and-white ones. With practice your visualization will improve, so for now go with what you have. Now, let's revisit the exercise, and mentally note any sounds that you might hear. Record your answers to these questions as before.

Type of sound?_____
(background noise, my inner voice commentating, etc.)

Volume of sound? _____
(loud, quiet, etc.)

Direction of sound?_____
(from the left, from the right, panoramic, etc.)

Brightness or dullness of sound?_____
(lifelike, muffled, etc.)

Quality of inner voice(s)?_____
(relaxed, focused, critical, encouraging, etc.)

By this point you'll know what types of image you make when you think about something you are certain you can do, and you know also what quality of sound is present, including any inner commentary. Finally, let's explore the feelings that are present. Close your eyes and run through the visualization again.

Where was the feeling strongest? _____
(e.g. stomach, chest, etc.)

What type of feeling was it?_____
(happiness, fear, excitement, etc.)

What texture did it have?_____
(tingly, spiky, smooth, etc.)

What temperature did it have? _____
(hot, cold, no temperature, etc.)

Was it a wide feeling or narrow?_____

Was it fast moving or slow?_____

How did the feeling move? _____
(upwards, downwards, clockwise, anti-clockwise)

How intense was the feeling?_____
(use a scale of 1–10)

We're going to call the above visualization *your picture of belief*. Many
of the exercises in this book will utilize this. How are we going to get
NLP working for you? We will get you believing in yourself, and your
ability to sleep.

Feel free to redo the above exercise until you feel really comfortable with
it. Change starts here. All you need to do is allow yourself an open mind.

FILL IN YOUR SLEEP DIARY

Let's put what we've learned to practical use. We're going to run
through a really simple visualization exercise that will programme
your mind to feel motivated when it comes to filling in your sleep
diary. These exercises make it much easier to complete tasks or
achieve goals.

Have a go

▶ This exercise is likely to take you 1–2 minutes.
▶ The best time to do it is just before you go to bed.

1 Close your eyes, and imagine you've just woken up in the
morning. See your sleep diary by the side of your bed (it doesn't
matter if you're currently unsure about filling it in; for this
exercise just pretend that you are).
2 How does it feel when you are motivated? Think about the
things in life you are motivated to do, and recall that motivated
feeling as strongly as you can. Then, in your mind's eye, picture
yourself filling in the diary.
3 Tell yourself, clearly: 'I want to fill in my sleep diary in the
morning!' As you do that, practise spinning the motivated feelings
around, as we learned to do before, so they become stronger.

4 Make changes to the mental movie in your mind's eye, adopting the look and feel of *your picture of belief*: the same level of colour, brightness, focus; the same location in your mind's eye, the same movement and the same sound.

5 Spin the motivated feelings around to make them stronger still. Keep imagining filling in the diary in a believable way. Make it feel like you're there.

6 Keep the images and the feelings going together for a minute or so, occasionally telling yourself, 'I want to fill in my sleep diary in the morning!'

This simple visualization exercise will build up a positive motivation to fill in your sleep diary. It is best to start using it when you have the materials (your sleep diary, a pen, the sign, etc.) in place. Do it each evening before you go to bed. It is quite straightforward, and good practice.

In the next chapter, we are going to introduce some changes to your sleeping environment. Remember the Neurological Levels Model we discussed in Chapter 2? The easiest place to start is usually our environment. We'll begin there and work our way up the levels systematically.

10 TIPS FOR SUCCESS

1 NLP is very much focused on *how* we do things. Your insomnia is not a random experience; the solution to it will reflect that.

2 By learning about sleep, your understanding of insomnia will be more accurate, and your efforts to overcome it will reflect that.

3 Sleep hygiene is a collection of changes that are designed to promote sleep. Using NLP techniques, we will aim to make it easy to implement these changes.

4 Anxiety is a common cause of insomnia. We will use NLP to help you overcome difficulties with anxious thoughts. If you can gain control of your thoughts and feelings, you can gain control of your sleep.

5 Relaxation helps to overcome insomnia. There are specific NLP techniques designed to help you feel drowsy, relaxed and ready to sleep.

6 Belief has a profound effect on our life. By freeing your mind of limiting beliefs, you make your recovery from insomnia much more likely.

7 Submodalities are the qualities of your sensory thoughts, e.g. picturing your loved one brightly and in colour, rather than dimly and in black-and-white.

8 Changing the submodalities of our thoughts changes our experience. For example, picturing images brightly can make our feelings stronger. Feelings can be taken and spun around, making them stronger or weaker.

9 You have a way of thinking about something that you are certain you can do well. We can examine the structure of your thoughts, and put that structure to good use. Positive change follows self-belief and certainty.

10 If you visualize using your sleep diary while generating strong feelings of motivation, you are much more likely to fill it in. Such exercises are the essence of NLP. This is your first step towards programming yourself for better sleep.

HOW AM I GETTING ON?

▶ *Have you looked at the various solutions we'll focus on in this book and decided which ones will be particularly helpful to you?*

▶ *Have you thought about a previous adversity in life, adversity that you have successfully overcome, and explored how you managed to overcome it?*

▶ *Have you practised the* submodality *exercises? We will use these types of exercise extensively as we go through our work together.*

▶ *Have you practised spinning feelings around in your body? This powerful technique can make all the difference to motivation, relaxation and anxiety.*

▶ *Have you completed the* picture of belief *exercise? This exercise is referred to repeatedly throughout this book. Your chances of success in overcoming sleeplessness will increase greatly if you complete this exercise to your satisfaction.*

▶ *Have you practised the exercise to fill in your sleep diary? If so, make sure you have the diary (and writing materials) to hand.*

Here is an excerpt from the previous chapter:

Without action, how can there be real learning? With that in mind, unless you can answer yes to at least three of the above questions, the best advice possible is to look again at the relevant parts of the chapter and do the exercises. Complete the exercises, and in time, everything can change.

At this stage, it's a point worth repeating.

4

Improving your sleeping environment

In this chapter you will learn:
- *about the power of conditioned responses*
- *how to optimize your sleeping environment for sleep*
- *how to get motivated to make the changes you need.*

> *A mind, like a home, is furnished by its owner.*
>
> Louis L'Amour

So far, we've learned about sleep and sleeplessness. We've learned about NLP and how to put it into action. It is time now to spend a bit less time discussing ideas and a bit more time making changes.

In Chapter 2 we noted that people learn best by actively acquiring, and applying, small chunks of knowledge. There is often a temptation to read books such as these without really acting on them, so we're going to take things a step at a time. As people, we can fear change. However, there is nothing to fear in change at your own pace. Change is best taken one step at a time.

In this chapter, we're going to focus on making your sleeping environment as conducive to sleep as possible.

Sleep hygiene and changes to your sleeping environment

If you recall, the Neurological Levels Model in Chapter 2 showed how you could look at different aspects of human beings: their identity, their values and beliefs, their skills and knowledge, their thoughts, feelings and behaviours, and their environment. These aspects are known as levels, and they interact with one another.

The Neurological Levels Model presents an organized framework within which to work. So, as we work through our programme to help you overcome insomnia, we will pay attention to each of these different levels. It is easiest to begin with the environment level. It will take only a day or so to optimize the sleeping conditions in your bedroom. To change a person's identity overnight is trickier, even with NLP!

You might ask, 'But why should I change my bedroom round? I like my life as it is!' Fine, but imagine if you had severe hay fever. Would you fill your house with flowers, making your nose itch all the time? If your work involved regular night shifts, would you buy a house next to a noisy school?

To overcome your insomnia, we will look at every angle possible. We're going to make small changes to your bedroom that have been demonstrated to help people sleep more easily. In some cases these small changes are all that is needed. For others, they make an important contribution to the overall picture. Overcoming insomnia is like most things: making several small changes with recovery emerging gradually.

The changes in this chapter relate to comfort and sleep hygiene. Sleep hygiene is mostly focused on the following piece of advice:

Make your bedroom comfortable, and use it only for sleep, reading this book or having sex.

If you have read about insomnia elsewhere, you will have seen this advice before. The human brain forms associations very quickly and very easily. Do you have a favourite chair? A food you associate with comfort? A song that really sets off the emotions? These are all examples of conditioning. To a given cue, we respond in a certain way. These types of association are incredibly powerful because they promote involuntary responses. We don't think about it, we just do it. (And of course this type of conditioning is used extensively in advertising!)

Back to insomnia: if you struggle to get to sleep in your bedroom, then you have developed a conditioned response. In response to the cue of getting into bed, your involuntary response is to be awake. Our goals with the following set of recommendations are:

- ▶ Make your bedroom a comfortable place to sleep.
- ▶ Break any negative conditioning between your bedroom and sleeplessness.

In the past, while in bed, you may have enjoyed watching TV, or reading, or surfing the internet. Unfortunately, things have changed. When things change, people have to adapt. You have developed a habit of sleeplessness in your bedroom. Your recovery now depends on adapting to this new set of circumstances.

In the next chapter we will look at your habits more thoroughly. For now, let's concentrate on making your bedroom an ideal place for sleep; the work we will do later will be much more effective when carried out in a comfortable environment that is free of negative conditioning. Taken together, these first steps, along with the exercises later in this book, will combine to create a comprehensive treatment programme for your insomnia. Making your bedroom an ideal place to sleep will help in many different ways, so let's take a look at the changes we can easily make.

REMOVE YOUR BEDSIDE CLOCK

Have you had that experience where, unable to sleep, you keep glancing at the time, counting down the hours? This is problematic in two ways. It is arousing behaviour: the anxiety created by sleepless clock-watching makes it more difficult to sleep. Second, over time, you are conditioning yourself to form negative associations between your bedroom and sleeplessness. Keeping your bedroom for only sleep or having sex breaks this negative conditioning. Clock-watching plays no part in sleeping, nor in making love (hopefully!).

Insight – clock-watching and insomnia

Our time is precious and we live busy lives. We need to be at work on time, back from our lunch break on time, back at home on time. Modern life is stressful and the clock plays a major part in that stress. Your bedroom should be a safe place where you can sleep easily. The best advice is to remove the bedside clock completely. Use your mobile phone as an alarm instead. At the very least, turn your clock away from your bed so you cannot see the time.

Insomnia sufferers tend to measure sleep in units of time, rather than units of quality. This way of thinking exacerbates insomnia in most people. If clock-watching is a major part of your insomnia, this recommendation is specifically for you.

REMOVE YOUR TV AND/OR COMPUTER

You possibly knew this piece of advice was coming. Again, this recommendation suggests that your bedroom should only be used for sleep, reading this book or having sex.

There are several problems with watching TV or using a computer in the bedroom. If you're watching your favourite box set or browsing the web, engaged and entertained, you will be stimulated, rather than relaxed. Even if you just watch something boring to help you doze off, behaviour that may have worked well in the past, now it just further reinforces the negative association between sleeplessness and your bedroom. Our brains form associations that are incredibly powerful. Here you're reinforcing a message to yourself, 'Even though I'm in my bedroom, I don't need to sleep!' This is not a great message to send to yourself if you have problems sleeping.

Something else worth noting. If you're watching TV in bed, there is a good chance that it is quite late. As we have mentioned before, sleep is driven, in part, by our body clock. Staying up late disrupts that clock. If your favourite programme is on late, then record it and watch it at a less disruptive time. Your problems with sleep have compelled you to read books on the matter; this means they're significant enough to begin making these small adjustments.

KEEP YOUR ROOM DARK AND QUIET

Is your room dark at night? It might seem obvious, but ensuring that your room is dark can be helpful. What are your curtains or blinds like? If the dawn light pours in, this isn't going to help, especially in cases of early-waking insomnia.

Assess the light situation in your bedroom realistically. Do the levels of light help or hinder your efforts to sleep? What steps can you take to address this? It could be that blackout blinds or curtains are the best option. As a last resort, some people use eye masks. Take an honest look at the levels of light in your room and ask, 'How can I improve this situation?'

The same can be said for noise. Trying to sleep in a noisy atmosphere is counter-productive. Unless you live in the countryside, external noise can be a problem. A person doesn't need complete silence to sleep and most people can tune out such noise. For those who struggle with insomnia, this skill can sometimes be lost. Noise is amplified via attention, causing anxiety, which then makes matters worse.

If you have noisy neighbours, it can be difficult to confront them in such situations, and it depends on your assessment of your neighbour's character. The most important point to remember here is that you have rights, and you needn't suffer noisy neighbours indefinitely. There are agencies you can approach, although the best advice would be to speak to them first, if their character allows it. Approach them calmly, reasonably, without emotion or accusation.

In approaching your neighbours, avoid putting them on the defensive. If they become defensive, it is unlikely they'll listen to your request. The goal is to get a reasonable agreement to curtail noise at bedtime. Your idea of bedtime might differ from theirs so compromise might be necessary. Ask them to turn TVs or stereos down, rather than off. Earplugs are an option and people get used to them. Another option is to use recordings, played on a low level, in your bedroom. Some people like recordings of natural sounds such as waves, forests and the like. White noise generators are also an option. Smartphones come with Apps that can aid sleep via relaxing noise.

Ultimately, there are some things we can control in life and some things we cannot. Later in this book we will try various relaxation exercises. Some of these will pay attention to blocking out background noise. For now, consider the levels of noise in your room. Is noise contributing to your difficulties in falling asleep? If so, how can you remedy the situation?

GIVE YOUR ROOM A SPRING CLEAN (AND KEEP IT CLEAN)

If your room is dusty, even moderately, then this can have a negative impact on your sleep. Breath, sleep and relaxation are inherently linked. If fluff and dust are genuinely a problem, and it pays to be honest with yourself here, then now is the time to do something about it. The same can be said for clutter. If clutter is an issue, then it's time for a clear-out. Your bedroom is not the place for piles of boxes, papers, discarded electronics equipment and the like. Aside from being a dust hazard, a cluttered room will not serve to relax you. Instead it will make you uncomfortable.

If you smoke, do you smoke in your bedroom? If so, the time has definitely come to consider smoking at the back door (or wherever), or at least in the living room. Smoking in your bedroom is a recipe for sleepless nights: stale air, inhaling secondary smoke, particles clogging up your airways. If you smoke in your bedroom, this one single change will significantly improve many aspects of your life.

In any bedroom, the greatest harbourer of dust is the bed itself. Would you consider your pillows and your mattress to be conducive to good sleep? Are they comfortable, and relatively new? Taking steps to remedy any problems here will make a difference, if you can afford the investment. Again, this isn't the whole story, but it is a significant part of it.

Cleaning your room, and keeping it clean, is an important part of what we are trying to achieve. Even if you're already fastidiously tidy, a good spring clean will help. Any negative associations will be weakened and that will count in your favour. These are not drastic steps. Making simple changes such as removing clocks and keeping your room comfortable really help.

If possible, stand in your sleeping environment now with fresh eyes. Take a look around, 360 degrees, and ask yourself, 'How, specifically, can I improve my bedroom so that it is clean, tidy and comfortable?'

KEEP YOUR ROOM AT THE RIGHT TEMPERATURE

Is your room too hot? Too cold? For some, it is difficult to keep the bedroom at the right temperature. People tend to prefer a cool bedroom, although this preference is not universal. Matters can be complicated when we share a bedroom with a partner who has different preferences.

It can be a puzzle, to an extent, to juggle these various factors. Sleeping with a window open can cool a room and improve airflow. Unfortunately, this can leave us susceptible to noise pollution. Experimenting with different duvets or blankets can help. If you are frequently waking up drenched in sweat, then your duvet's tog rating is too high. If you're waking up and you're shivering, then consider an extra blanket. People with insomnia often have the problem of feeling too chilly; a tightening of blood vessels in the skin reduces blood flow, causing feelings of being too cold. A draught excluder can also help with this.

If you find yourself too hot in bed, a cooling shower beforehand can help. Cooling though, not freezing! Taking a shower before bed can be relaxing as well.

CHECKLIST FOR OPTIMIZING YOUR SLEEPING ENVIRONMENT

Let's create a really simple checklist of things to do. You won't necessarily need to do all of these things, but be honest in your appraisal of what does need doing. The key actions here are: remove your clock, TV and computer; de-clutter your room and thoroughly clean it; remove ashtrays if you smoke in there; and consider a new pillow and mattress, or at least get the right duvet for your preferred temperature. Speak to your neighbours, or buy earplugs, if external noise is a problem. Consider heavier curtains or blinds if light is a problem.

Making these changes will help some people overcome their insomnia straight away. Our environment impacts on our behaviour, and there is clear evidence that sleep hygiene works. Given the misery insomnia creates, perhaps the time has come to give this a thorough try.

Strongly recommended changes:

▶ Remove ashtrays.
▶ Remove your bedside clock.
▶ Remove your TV. *(Do you need a drill, or help, to remove the TV bracket?)*
▶ Remove your computer.
▶ De-clutter your room.
▶ Clean your room thoroughly.

Optional changes, if required:

▶ Buy earplugs.
▶ Buy a gel eyemask.
▶ Buy a draught excluder.
▶ Buy a new duvet.
▶ Purchase blinds/curtains.
▶ Buy a new mattress and pillows.
▶ Speak to the neighbours.

Overcoming obstacles to change

How do you feel about these changes? Some people will feel motivated straight away. These changes are logical and logic can be enough. For some, there will be resistance and reluctance. Let's go through any objections you might have, and come up with exercises that will help.

A RELUCTANCE TO ASK ONE'S PARTNER

In some instances, a person may be reluctant to discuss these changes with their partner. If you share your bedroom with a fellow smoker, or somebody who likes to watch TV in bed, you might prefer to avoid discussing such changes, for fear of causing an argument. However, the reality is that these recommendations are simple and will not cause too much disruption to anyone.

....
Insight – co-operation within the family
Co-operation within the family doesn't always happen, but just as with your neighbours, if you approach them in the spirit of compromise, and are willing to put aside squabbles and be pragmatic, there is a good chance that your partner will agree to the recommended improvements presented in this book.

Put it into perspective, and your partner, ultimately, should be on your side. Is removing a clock or TV really too much to ask when a person's stress levels, and potentially their health, are being directly affected?
....

A FEAR OF CHANGE, FAILURE AND SUCCESS

As people, we tend to fear or dislike change. Familiarity suits us, whereas the unknown can frighten us. A fear or dislike of change could make you look at these simple changes and feel reluctant. You could then think thoughts such as:

▶ *I don't have enough time to move my computer, or de-clutter my room, or buy a duvet, or whichever.*
▶ *I will make these changes, but I'll do it at some point in the future.*
▶ *I can't move my TV or computer, I have nowhere to put them.*
▶ *I can't de-clutter my room; it's too much effort or too complicated.*
▶ *I want to keep things as they are, I'll learn to sleep another way.*
▶ *I hate moving things around; I'll just read the rest of the book!*

- ▶ *I don't need to do this bit; I'll skip on to the next.*
- ▶ *This doesn't count for me, just for other people whose insomnia is really bad.*

Perhaps you can recognize some of these thoughts? They sound plausible and may contain nuggets of truth. On closer inspection, they do not seem rational. Not enough time? How much time would you need? An hour or two, at the most. Avoiding making the changes recommended in this chapter will contribute to your struggles with sleeplessness.

As humans, we tend to like what is familiar. Familiarity is comfortable. We also tend to be excellent procrastinators, putting things off where action would be a more logical course of action. How many times have you said to yourself, 'I'll start that diet on Monday', or 'I'll start work on that report tomorrow', or 'I'll sort out that cupboard some day'? In reality, we're trading discomforts here. There is discomfort involved in needing to diet or needing to write a report, but there is discomfort involved in actually dieting, or actually writing a report. Faced with the choice of two types of discomfort, we choose what seems to be the lesser of the two: to put things off. Stagnation then follows.

Sometimes, we fear failure. What if the recommendations in this book don't work? That thought can create a reluctance to act, which then causes a failure to change. Remember the NLP presupposition, 'there is no failure, only feedback'? If you put in place these changes, and they don't pay off initially, then we will look to further changes in this book. Combined, all of these changes will add up to your best chance of success. A fear of failure is the least rational reason to avoid acting in your best interests.

When you think about putting these recommendations into action, do you feel resistant, reluctant or inert? Uncomfortable, or even fearful? If so, you are thinking emotionally, rather than logically. If there is such a thing as failure, it looks like inaction. You were motivated to buy this book. Now, realize:

Acting on these recommendations will help to change your life – you can do it!

Whatever your experience of insomnia, it can be improved. With the following exercise, we'll put in place the motivation to get started.

Have a go

▶ This exercise is likely to take 1–2 minutes.

▶ If you need to, review your answers to *your picture of belief* exercise in Chapter 3, and refresh your memory as to what it looks and feels like.

▶ Repeat this exercise as many times as you need up until the date(s) you set.

▶ Really get into it, and be creative!

1 First, set a date for when you're going to:
    a make simple changes, such as removing clocks:_____
    (you could do this today)
    b make any required purchases, such as duvets:_____
    c make any major changes, such as de-cluttering:_____
    (weekends work well for this)

2 Think of how much you want to be able to get a good night's sleep in a comfy, clean, restful room, free from distractions, free from noise. In your mind's eye, watch yourself sleeping, clearly happy in bed. Make this image as bright and colourful as you can.

3 Imagine being in the room, watching yourself. Enjoy the clean, comfortable nature of the room around you. Really get into this until you feel powerfully motivated to make your room as clean and comfortable as possible. Think about how much you want better sleep.

4 Take those feelings of motivation and spin them around your body (as we practised in Chapter 3). Make them stronger and stronger.

5 Imagine yourself making the required changes: removing ashtrays and bedside clocks, de-cluttering your room and cleaning it; keep those motivated feelings spinning around. Imagine yourself cleaning and feeling really satisfied by such positive change: removing your TV, moving your computer, even putting up blinds or curtains if required. Make these pictures similar to your *picture of belief* in look and feel (see Chapter 3).

6 All the while, keep those positive, motivated feelings spinning around, amplifying them so they become as strong as they can.

7 Finally, picture your clean, comfortable, calming room and state to yourself, '*I want this!*'

Practise this exercise, memorizing the steps, until you can make it a smooth experience. The most important part is the feelings. Aim to get strong feelings of motivation fizzing around your body. The stronger the feelings, the stronger your drive to move forward. You can do it!

PUTTING IT ALL TOGETHER

We have a list of helpful changes to put in place: adjustments to your sleeping environment that will make it a comfortable, relaxing place to be; where only positive associations are created, and old, negative associations are gradually erased. You have an exercise to help you put these changes in place, and a good deal of reasoning as to why these changes will contribute towards your freedom from insomnia.

The recommendations in this chapter are in preparation for what comes next. In Chapter 5 we will look at positive changes we can make to your behaviour. Changes that will mean you take a huge step forward as you reconnect with your natural ability to sleep.

10 TIPS FOR SUCCESS

1 Your bedroom should be used for three things only: sleeping, reading this book and having sex. This might seem strict, but there is enough research to back this claim for you to act upon it. It will make a huge difference to your life.

2 Smoking, watching the clock, watching TV or surfing the 'net will only exacerbate your insomnia. These activities programme your brain to think, '*I don't have to sleep in my bedroom*'. That is a really unhelpful suggestion for somebody who struggles to get to sleep.

3 Keeping your room dark and quiet helps tremendously. Where possible, explore putting up black-out blinds or curtains, and speaking with noisy neighbours, in order to make your sleeping environment as comfortable as possible.

4 Keeping your room clean and clutter-free will also go a long way to improving your sleep. Time for a spring clean.

5 Ensuring you are the right temperature in bed can make all the difference. Explore different ways in which you can sleep at the temperature which best suits you.

6 We sometimes fear change and failure. Sometimes we just dislike the discomfort of doing things, but these are not rational reasons to suffer from your insomnia any longer.

7 We sometimes procrastinate, putting things off when acting would be best. Putting off the recommendations in this book will contribute to further sleeplessness, whereas acting will make a positive difference!

8 If there is such a thing as failure, then it looks like inaction.

9 Use the exercise to optimize your sleep environment as frequently as you need to so that you put those changes in place. You can do it!

10 The recommendations in this chapter will make your bedroom a comfortable, relaxing place to be; positive associations will be created, and negative associations are gradually erased.

HOW AM I GETTING ON?

▶ *Have you been through the list of recommended changes to make to your bedroom, deciding on which ones are appropriate for you?*

▶ *If appropriate, have you spoken with your partner or spouse? Get them on board to help you make the changes you need to make.*

▶ *Have you used the exercise to* optimize your sleep environment, *several times, in order to get going?*

▶ *Have you set a date to make the required changes to your bedroom? These recommendations will help you change your life and should be made before carrying on with this book. You can do it!*

Freedom from insomnia is in your hands. It is the job of any therapist, coach or author to help people connect with their own inner strengths and capabilities. You're reading this book because you want to overcome your difficulties with sleeplessness. Ensuring that you can answer yes to the above questions will give you the best chance of success. What can you do to make that happen now?

5

....

Increasing your drive to sleep

In this chapter you will learn:
- *about behaviours that promote sleep*
- *how a regular routine can help beat insomnia*
- *how these recommendations work in real life*
- *how to become more determined.*

> *After years of studying sleep, one of the sure things known about sleep deprivation is that it makes you sleepy.*
>
> Dr Wilse Webb

In the previous chapter we discussed how using your bedroom solely for the purpose of sleeping, reading this book or having sex will help to break any negative conditioning acquired as a result of your insomnia. We then put in place some changes designed to break that conditioning and make your bedroom an ideal place to sleep. Before proceeding, have you acted on those recommendations? Are you happy with the result?

Behaviours that promote sleep

Now that your bedroom is an ideal place to sleep, let's look at those behaviours that will help you to overcome insomnia. The recommendations in this chapter are designed with one of three goals in mind:

▶ To reset your body clock, so the circadian process functions normally.
▶ To allow sleep pressure, the drive created by the homeostatic process, to build during the day.

▶ To break any negative associations between your bedroom and sleep, replacing them instead with positive associations.

The recommendations in this chapter are very straightforward – simple changes to your day-to-day routine that will increase the likelihood of sleep:

▶ Establish a regular waking time each day, including weekends, and rise within 10 minutes of waking.
▶ Seek out natural daylight as early as possible after rising.
▶ Avoid caffeinated drinks, food, nicotine and vigorous exercise after certain times.
▶ If you don't typically exercise, strongly consider going for an evening stroll or walking the dog, tai chi or relaxing yoga; just for 20 minutes in the evening.
▶ Avoid daytime napping.
▶ Become just a bit more active.
▶ Undertake a relaxing activity before bed.
▶ Avoid going to bed before your preferred bedtime, and even then only go to bed when sleepy.
▶ Use your bedroom only for sleeping, reading this book or having sex; avoid watching TV, worrying, clock-watching and especially *trying* to get to sleep.
▶ If you don't fall asleep within 20 minutes of turning off the lights, get up and do something else; this also counts when you wake up for the last time in the morning.

Let's go through each recommendation in more detail and explain the rationale behind each one.

ESTABLISH A REGULAR WAKING TIME EACH DAY, INCLUDING WEEKENDS, AND RISE WITHIN 10 MINUTES OF WAKING

In Chapter 1, we discussed the two systems that drive sleep: the circadian process and the homeostatic process. When functioning correctly, these two independent systems combine and sleep comes easily.

Having an irregular rising time causes problems for both systems. Where our body clock works well, the circadian process will produce a drive to sleep at around 11 p.m. Any behaviour that interferes with the body clock's natural timing will interfere with the circadian-dependent drive to sleep. Having a regular rising time keeps our body clock ticking over nicely; an irregular rising time weakens it.

As mentioned in Chapter 1, our body's homeostatic process increases the pressure we feel to sleep. This pressure increases with each hour spent awake. If a person rises considerably later one day, there is less time for sleep pressure to build, and they will not feel tired that night. Rising at a set point, relatively early each day, means there will be ample time for the body to feel sleepy. Consistency is key, with sleep as with many things in life.

What about weekends? If we were to be strict, the recommendation would be to stick to your rising time, even on Saturday and Sunday. For many of us, that isn't likely to happen. So compromise. At the weekend, if you'd prefer to sleep in, try a difference of 60–90 minutes maximum, ideally just 60.

Getting out of bed within 10 minutes of waking also helps. It is not good to associate your bed with wakefulness, even relaxed or drowsy wakefulness. Place your alarm away from your bed so you need to get up to switch it off. Then, fill in your sleep diary, take a shower and soak up some daylight. It is typical to experience grogginess for the first 30 minutes after waking. However, you will be up and your body clock will be ticking.

If you are having problems sleeping, there is a good chance that you will be tired in the morning. For some, it can seem as if wild horses would fail to drag them from their beds! Sticking to a regular rising time is such an important recommendation. Enlist the help of your partner, or your friends, or your colleagues, even your boss! Later in this book, you'll be given an exercise that will help. For now, consider how much you'd like to overcome your insomnia. Following this recommendation is a big step in the right direction. Choose a regular rising time that suits you and set your alarm today.

SEEK OUT NATURAL DAYLIGHT AS SOON AS POSSIBLE AFTER RISING

Our body clock is sensitive to light. Upon rising, fill in your sleep diary, shower and seek out some daylight as quickly as possible. Open the curtains, go to the kitchen door and drink a cup of coffee as you watch the sky slowly brighten. Work this into your morning routine. You're starting a countdown, telling your body clock, 'OK, I will go to sleep in 16 hours and counting.'

AVOID CAFFEINATED DRINKS, FOOD, NICOTINE AND EXERCISE AFTER CERTAIN TIMES

This recommendation focuses on those behaviours that override the body's sleep-promoting systems. Most people recognize coffee as a stimulant. Coffee contains caffeine, as do other drinks such as tea, carbonated soft drinks, energy drinks and the like. After 3 p.m., switch from caffeinated drinks to something caffeine-free. Learning to love water is always a fantastic idea. In time, a person can get used to anything. Even herbal teas!

When it comes to coffee, be honest with yourself. You understand that you are having sleep problems, so if you drink too much coffee, or you continue to drink coffee throughout the day, ask yourself, 'How is this helping?' If your sleep problems are making you miserable, is that misery worth the extra cup of coffee?

It is always a good idea to eat healthily, and eating healthily can aid sleep. Whatever your diet, avoid consuming food within three hours of your bedtime. So, if you aim to be asleep by 11.30 p.m., eat no later than 8.30 p.m. Where possible, keep to a regular eating time in the evening and try to prioritize healthier, non-processed foods over processed foods. Processed foods invariably contain a lot of sugar, and sugar is not going to help you sleep.

Insight – advice for smokers

If you smoke, you might find it a relaxing experience. Unfortunately, nicotine is also a stimulant. If you're trying to get a good night's sleep, a stimulant is the last thing you need before bed. Instead, try to make your last cigarette around 45–60 minutes before you go to bed. As you will know, smoking is habit-forming! Within a couple of days, this new time will feel natural.

In Chapter 9 there is an exercise that can help with this. For now, see how you get on. If you feel that excessive smoking is contributing to your insomnia, then give serious consideration to using a 'quit smoking' service. It is not just your sleep that will improve.

Perhaps you enjoy regular, vigorous exercise? If so, ensure that you finish your exercising at least three hours before your bedtime. Exercise aids sleep and it's a really good idea to get some. If you don't exercise, now would be a good time to start! This does not have to mean vigorous exercise: go for a stroll, learn some tai chi or relaxing yoga. Even 20 minutes of housework will help. Taking gentle to moderate exercise in the evening will help you overcome insomnia. You can take gentle exercise at any point in the evening.

In summary:

▶ Avoid drinking caffeinated drinks after 3 p.m.
▶ Eat at a regular time, no later than three hours before going to sleep.
▶ Avoid smoking later than 45–60 minutes before going to sleep.
▶ Avoid vigorous exercise later than three hours before going to sleep.

With these recommendations, it is a question of timing.

AVOID DAYTIME NAPPING

Insomnia doesn't usually lead to daytime sleepiness, although it does create a fixation on feeling fatigued and therefore desiring sleep. If you feel tired in the afternoon, and you have the option, the temptation is to take a nap. For the next three months avoid daytime napping if possible. Taking a nap will interfere with your drive to sleep that night. The homeostatic process, rather than building sleep pressure, will instead be reduced. This will then reduce the likelihood of falling asleep at your preferred bedtime.

Instead, drink a refreshing warm drink. Caffeine is fine if it is before 3 p.m. Then go for a brisk walk. Take 20 minutes or so to do something stimulating. Within 20 minutes, the desire to nap will have passed. You may still feel fatigued, and you may still feel that you would like to sleep, but these two experiences will not cause you to actually fall asleep. Avoiding napping will make such a difference to your chances of sleep at bedtime.

BECOME JUST A BIT MORE ACTIVE

How active are you during the day? In this modern age we live sedentary lifestyles that contribute to insomnia, among other things. Even simply walking more can help. What would happen if you got off the bus a stop earlier and walked? If you took the train rather than the car, or if you did a little more around the house? Exercise helps people overcome insomnia and there are small changes that could easily fit into your life.

UNDERTAKE A RELAXING ACTIVITY BEFORE BED

Imagine if, at 11.30 p.m., you were working on a presentation for work the next day. You want to be in bed by midnight (*'I must get some sleep, I have a big day tomorrow!'*). So, instead of relaxing and priming yourself for sleep, you're anxiously rewriting your presentation, thinking hard, getting stressed. Ideal preparation? Of course not. Before sleep, it helps if you wind down and allow yourself to relax.

For around 30–60 minutes before bed, switch off the TV, put away any work and spend some time relaxing. In general terms, this means avoiding activities that involve a screen, so surfing the internet is best avoided. Some people find reading quite stimulating, whereas others find it relaxing. Non-fiction, including this book, should be fine. Practising the exercises in this book would be a good idea. Anything that will help you slow down, and relax.

For some, a warm shower helps. If you have problems with feeling too hot or cold during the night, take that into consideration and choose the temperature of your shower accordingly. As mentioned previously, exercises such as tai chi and some of the more relaxing types of yoga are particularly good. Anything that will not stress you. Anything that helps you to relax.

As with all things, repetition is key: having a fixed evening routine where you've eaten, you've watched some TV, you've relaxed and let things quieten down, and then you've retired to bed. With a regular routine you are conditioning yourself to sleep on cue.

AVOID GOING TO BED BEFORE YOUR PREFERRED BEDTIME, AND EVEN THEN ONLY GO TO BED WHEN SLEEPY

Having a fixed bedtime, and not going to bed before that bedtime (even if you feel sleepy), serves a very important purpose. Going to bed earlier than your preferred bedtime interferes with your body clock and strengthens negative conditioning. This is to be avoided.

Insight – early nights can lead to fractured sleep

In Chapter 1 we discussed the various stages of sleep. The deeper, non-REM sleep is broken into four stages. Stages 1 and 2 are characterized by the relaxation of the body. Sleep then deepens further. Stages 3 and 4 are when the body's restorative processes unfold. This deep sleep is our ultimate goal.

When you retire before your normal bedtime, instead of getting the right amount of slow-wave sleep, you're likely to get too much Stage 1 and 2 sleep, coupled with an increase in REM sleep. The reasons for this are not fully understood, but insomnia sufferers frequently find their sleep shallow and fragmented. Going to bed earlier than your preferred bedtime creates problems for your body clock *and* your sleep quality.

Remember, we are aiming to increase the amount of quality sleep that you get. This means working with your body's natural processes. Going to bed at your preferred bedtime, even if you are tired beforehand, helps to keep your body clock in order, and you will gently phase into deep, slow-wave sleep naturally. Six hours of quality sleep, including the right amount of slow-wave sleep, is better than eight hours of fragmented, shallow sleep. Going to bed before your preferred bedtime interferes with the process of getting deep, restorative, slow-wave sleep. If you don't have a regular, preferred bedtime, now is a great time to decide on one.

If your bedtime comes and goes, and you're just not sleepy, the only thing to do is wait until you are. Take this book, sit away from your bedroom and read. Practise the exercises, particularly those in Chapter 7. For some, staying up can feel counter-intuitive or even frightening: *'But I'll feel terrible in the morning if I stay up until 3 a.m. reading this damned book!'* It is true that staying up late and sticking to your regular rising time will leave you tired and fatigued. Lying in bed awake will also leave you feeling tired and fatigued the next day. Plus, it will strengthen your insomnia, for all of the reasons we have discussed. It is incorrect to think that lying in bed, trying to get to sleep, is the next best thing to sleep. That is a myth. If you only go to bed when sleepy, even if it is late, you'll find that you begin to fall asleep more and more quickly, and your insomnia will begin to change.

So, if you're not sleepy, and even if it is several hours past your preferred bedtime, stay up and practise the exercises in this book. In time, your sleep systems will reset themselves.

USE YOUR BEDROOM ONLY FOR SLEEPING, READING THIS BOOK OR HAVING SEX; AVOID WATCHING TV, WORRYING, CLOCK WATCHING AND ESPECIALLY TRYING TO GET TO SLEEP

We have spoken about the ease with which associations form. We want to avoid associating your bed with wakefulness. Using your bedroom only for sleeping, reading this book or having sex is important. It will help to dismantle any negative associations acquired as a result of your insomnia, allowing you to build positive associations instead. It is easy to read or watch TV elsewhere. And this recommendation does help many people.

From this point on, let's be strict about these matters. This is a comprehensive list of what can be done in your bedroom:

- ▶ Waking up in the morning.
- ▶ Filling in your sleep diary when you get out of bed.
- ▶ Dressing, doing your hair, etc.
- ▶ Going to bed.
- ▶ Having sex.
- ▶ Reading this book or listening to the MP3 (enhanced e-book version).
- ▶ Relaxing and going to sleep.

Let's look at a list of things to avoid while in your bedroom:

- ▶ Watching the clock.
- ▶ Watching TV.
- ▶ Surfing the internet or playing games (if you must use your computer in your bedroom, certainly do not use it while you are actually in bed).
- ▶ Fiddling with your phone.
- ▶ Reading novels.
- ▶ Drawing, studying, cartography (!) and the like.
- ▶ Worrying, planning or solving problems.
- ▶ Eating.
- ▶ Arguing.
- ▶ Having long lie-ins where you lie there doing nothing.
- ▶ Spending time in bed *trying* to get to sleep.

Now is the time to be strict with yourself. Each of these activities hinders your chances of finding deep, restful sleep. Whatever attachment you might have to them, is insomnia a price worth paying? If you feel like eating, eat in another room. If you are arguing with your spouse, break off the argument and move to another room.

And if you're lying in bed, tossing and turning, trying to get to sleep? The early hours can bring troubling thoughts. With nothing to do other than lie and think, our minds turn to those things that we need to resolve or that concern us in some way. *This includes worrying about sleep and insomnia*. Your thoughts racing, turning around and around. From what we have learned so far about sleep, and about conditioning, clearly such experiences are to be avoided. This leads us on to our next recommendation.

IF YOU DON'T FALL ASLEEP WITHIN 20 MINUTES OF TURNING OFF THE LIGHTS, GET UP AND DO SOMETHING ELSE

This also counts when you wake up for the last time in the morning. To avoid wakefulness in bed, if you cannot fall asleep, then get up, leave the bedroom, sit comfortably somewhere and practise the exercises in this book, particularly in Chapter 7. Spend 30 minutes or so, and then try going back to bed. Spending time in bed awake will only make your insomnia worse.

This is also true for waking during the night or in the early morning hours. So, should you wake at 4.30 a.m. one morning, and after 20 minutes or so it is clear that you are not going to fall back to sleep, then the best thing to do is get up and read this book. After 30 minutes or so, try going back to bed.

Insight – when your bedroom is your only room

For some, getting up and leaving the bedroom is not always possible. If you live in student accommodation or a bedsit, you will have little choice but to spend a lot of time awake in your sleeping space. This can be problematic.

In such circumstances, keep a desk and chair in your room and make use of them. Avoid using your bed for anything other than sleep, having sex, or reading this book (so no study, no watching TV, no surfing the 'net). At night, if you find that you don't fall asleep within 20 minutes of turning off the lights, get out of bed and practise the exercises in this book. This way you'll avoid forming negative associations between your bed and sleeplessness.

The point of these recommendations is to build up a regular routine; a time for awakening, a time for exercising, a time for eating, a time for relaxing and a time for sleeping. When you have a regular time for such things, your body clock becomes stronger and you will sleep better. How does this work in practice? Let's take a thorough look at a case study, so that we can see how these recommendations contribute to beating insomnia.

A case study in behaviours that promote sleep

Denise, 44, was a typical insomnia sufferer. She had a stressful job as a financial controller in a medium-sized business. Married for 20 years, her family was financially comfortable, but that had not always been the case. Her marriage had been through its fair share of difficulty, but was fundamentally strong. Several years ago, she'd lost a very close friend to illness, and her insomnia started then.

Although her grief had eventually subsided, her insomnia was still causing a great deal of misery in her life.

Denise suffered from sleep onset insomnia and sleep maintenance insomnia. Often she would lie in bed for around 90–120 minutes before falling asleep; sleep was then fractured, waking two or three times per night. She would also wake up too early in the morning, finding that she could rarely get back to sleep. Her husband was supportive, for the most part, but having never had sleeping difficulties himself, he couldn't fully understand the extent of Denise's problem.

Denise's weekday routine involved arriving at work for 8.30 a.m., with no real lunch break, and regular cups of tea or coffee throughout the day. At home she would eat at a reasonable hour, and then watch TV before going to bed at around 10 p.m. Sometimes she would nap for an hour or so after dinner, but this was rare. On getting into bed, she would read until around 11.30 p.m., when her husband would join her and they'd switch out the lights. Denise would then lie there until finally falling asleep at around 1.30 a.m. She would always be out of bed by 6.30 a.m., often after spending an hour or so awake in bed. Denise regularly felt that she hadn't slept a wink, and would complain to others that she barely slept. When questioned, she consistently rated the quality of her sleep as very poor.

During the day, Denise felt tired and irritable, and that her performance in work was significantly impaired. She constantly ached and, on occasion, felt sleepy in the afternoons. She often cancelled social engagements because of her tiredness. Her thoughts regularly turned to sleep, and how to get more of it. At weekends she would usually wake at around 6 a.m., and then stay in bed until 8 a.m., when she'd typically fall back to sleep. Denise felt anxious about going to bed on most nights, and this would be most pronounced on Sunday evenings. Sunday nights were the most difficult, sleep-wise, and it would not be unusual for her to still be awake at 1.30 a.m.

Here are the changes it was recommended for Denise to make:

- ▶ Remove her bedside clock.
- ▶ Remove the TV from her bedroom.
- ▶ Get up at 6.30 a.m. each day; if she woke earlier, and could not get to sleep within 25 minutes, then rise at that time.
- ▶ Avoid tea or coffee after 3 p.m.
- ▶ Try to be more active each day.

- Try a tai chi DVD in the evenings, just for 20 minutes.
- Have a 30-minute period of relaxing before bed.
- Avoid going to bed before her preferred bedtime, and even then only go to bed when sleepy.
- If she didn't fall asleep within 20 minutes after turning off the lights, get up and do something else. This was also true when she woke up in the night.

At first Denise was dubious about making changes to her sleeping environment, and her husband wasn't pleased at the idea of removing the TV from the bedroom! However, with some talking he agreed to watch the TV downstairs instead. She was also reluctant to remove her bedside clock, although she did acknowledge that clock-watching played a big part in her insomnia, and found that she easily adapted to using the alarm on her mobile phone instead. Other than that, Denise's bedroom was comfortable, clean and dark at night.

Making the change of getting up at 6.30 a.m. was easy for Denise. Sometimes she would wake earlier than the desired time, and it was with some reluctance that she got out of bed at 5.30 a.m. Denise found that she could easily stop drinking coffee at 3 p.m. Like many office workers, Denise didn't have a lunch break to speak of, and normally ate at her desk. Instead, as recommended, she started leaving the office for 20 minutes, going for a walk and getting a bit of fresh air.

Denise tried tai chi, but found it wasn't for her. However, she did enjoy taking a warm shower in the evening after dinner; it did not seem like too much of a commitment, and she found it relaxing. The first couple of days reading downstairs, rather than in bed, felt really quite strange and she missed the comfort of bed. Again, this was something she got used to quite quickly. After reading, Denise would practise some relaxation exercises, and stuck to this quite well.

The most difficult change Denise was advised to make centred on bedtime. She would frequently feel fatigued by 10.30 p.m., but not sleepy. Often she would go to bed, only to get up some 20 minutes later. At first this made her anxious, and she fretted about feeling tired the next day. However, with the (sometimes gruff) support of her husband, she would get up, go downstairs, and practise various relaxation exercises. Normally, she would be back in bed within the hour and, over the course of a week or so, found that she was going to sleep more and more quickly each night.

It is true to say that Denise found the days quite tough to begin with, and on many occasions would yearn to go to bed before her preferred bedtime of 10 p.m. However, with support, and a commitment to change, she resisted that temptation and stayed up at least until her bedtime; later on those days where she recognized that, although tired, she wasn't drowsy enough to actually sleep at any point soon. Difficult, but not unmanageable, and her body clock readjusted itself in a relatively short space of time.

At first this change wasn't consistent. Some nights were really good, but on other nights Denise would struggle and she felt quite frustrated. It still felt quite strange to get out of bed, but with time she started to understand that lying in bed (trying to get to sleep) hadn't really helped her in the past. Gradually, her ability to get to sleep improved: after three or four weeks Denise would fall asleep within 25 minutes of going to bed on most nights. Denise found that taking a shower, and practising with the relaxation exercises, had really helped.

Denise wasn't spending much more time asleep. Perhaps an hour or so each night. Rather, she was finding that her sleep was much deeper. She still woke up early in the morning, but with the relaxation exercises she had practised, coupled with less anxiety, Denise found that she could actually go back to sleep on most occasions. After two months or so she was sleeping much more soundly. She felt more refreshed each day, and was encouraged that her situation was improving.

Insight – Denise's challenge

In Denise's case we can see that her two big difficulties were staying awake until her preferred bedtime, and staying up beyond her bedtime on those occasions when she knew that she wouldn't fall asleep easily. This was her challenge: the hurdle that needed to be overcome for things to improve. This is often the nature of change. There are difficulties that we must move beyond in order to get what we want. To overcome your insomnia, in reality, will require a period of focus, determination and desire.

The following exercise will help you to build the required motivation and determination to act on the recommendations in this book. It could help with staying up until your preferred bedtime, or taking light exercise, or getting up if you don't fall asleep immediately. Use it often, and use it when required. This exercise can also be used at night to help you get out of bed in the morning.

Have a go

▶ This exercise is likely to take just 1–2 minutes.
▶ Repeat it as often as you need.
▶ The best time to use this exercise is when you need it.
▶ As you perform the exercise, relax your shoulders, your eyes, and allow yourself to be comfortable.

1 Close your eyes, and imagine – how nice would it feel to have deeper sleep? Think about the peace, the rest, and allow yourself to feel good about it. Then think about what you need to feel determined about; for example, staying up until your preferred bedtime, even if you're tired.

2 Think about how you really want to be able to sleep more easily, and how staying up until your preferred bedtime will help. Imagine the good quality sleep you will get, in really vivid detail, and feel determined to carry the recommendation through.

3 Make the feelings of determination stronger by spinning them through your body.

4 Imagine yourself, as if you were watching yourself on TV, staying up until your bedtime (or whichever scenario you are building up determination to complete) while spinning the motivated feelings around. Make them stronger and stronger still.

5 Then, step into your body, so you're looking out through your own eyes, *in the television screen as it were*, and replay the scenario again, keeping the feelings of determination spinning around your body. Tell yourself, in a clear, determined voice, 'I am doing this so I can sleep better!'

BECOME MORE DETERMINED

You can use this exercise to become more determined in the moment, or you can use it to programme yourself to do something at a later time. To use this exercise to get out of bed, complete it three times before going to bed. If on waking you still feel seduced by the idea of comfortably lying in bed, use the exercise again. With a little practice, your determination levels will continue to improve.

Without determination there can only be stagnation. Determination is the drive to act, and it is via action that things really change. You *can* put in place the recommendations in this book. You *can* overcome your insomnia. Realize there is nothing stopping you from making the changes you desire. Sometimes, we just need to relearn how to unleash our determination to carry things through.

Consider how good it would feel to leave behind your difficulties with insomnia. With that in mind, resolve to use this exercise daily. With determination, your life can change in innumerable ways. And how good would that feel?

10 TIPS FOR SUCCESS

1 Your behaviour affects your sleep. You can strengthen your body clock, your drive to sleep, and your positive associations between your bed and sleep just by making a few simple changes to your day-to-day routine.

2 Have a regular waking time each day, and rise within 10 minutes of waking. Then, seek out daylight as early as possible. This will help to set your body clock and build sleep pressure.

3 Avoid caffeinated drinks, food, nicotine and exercise after certain times. These are all stimulants that interfere with your body's drive to sleep.

4 Avoid daytime napping. Napping interferes with your drive to sleep; it will cause problems later that night.

5 Instead, try to be a bit more active during the day. Even a little extra walking can help. In the evening, gentle exercise for 20 minutes will increase your drive to sleep.

6 Undertake a relaxing activity in the evening for a period before bed. This will help you wind down, so avoid anything overly stimulating. Reading non-fiction, taking a shower, walking the dog, or gentle exercise such as tai chi can all help.

7 Avoid going to bed before your preferred bedtime, and even then only go to bed when sleepy. Sleeping before your preferred bedtime will affect your body clock and interfere with your sleep. Going to bed when you don't feel sleepy promotes the association between your bed and wakefulness, which is to be avoided at all costs.

8 If you don't fall asleep within 20 minutes of turning off the lights, get up, and practise the exercises in this book. This also counts when you wake up in the night or in the early morning. Lying in bed trying to get to sleep does not help in any way.

9 Behaviours that beat insomnia are all about timing. Aim to get a bit of a routine going; probably the most important

recommendations in this book are to decide on a regular rising time and a regular bedtime, and to stick to them.

10 Change requires determination. You can build determination to do anything. Practise the exercise to become more determined, and you'll find the changes in this book are easy to implement.

HOW AM I GETTING ON?

▶ *Have you decided on a regular rising time? Have you decided on a regular bedtime? If so, set your alarm and stick to them!*

▶ *What could you do in the morning that would expose you to daylight? An early morning stroll? A cup of coffee at the kitchen door? Early morning sunlight will help set your body clock for an earlier bedtime.*

▶ *Have you reviewed the timing of stimulants such as caffeinated drinks, vigorous exercise, your evening meal and, if relevant, your last cigarette? By what time should you avoid each of these activities?*

▶ *Have you thought about how you could, if necessary, inject a little more activity into your life? Aim to walk more.*

▶ *What relaxing activities could you enjoy in the evening before bed? It could be something passive, such as reading (non-fiction may be best), or gently active such as tai chi. What would suit you?*

▶ *Have you practised the exercise to become more determined? What results did you get?*

▶ *Have you understood that lying in bed doing anything other than sleeping is counter-productive? Whether you have just retired to bed or whether you have awoken in the night or early morning, if you have been awake in bed for 20 minutes, then it is always best to get up, and do something else.*

How you behave impacts on how you sleep. An extreme, obvious example would be to try to sleep after 15 cups of coffee. Conventional wisdom tells us that drinking so much coffee is only going to keep you awake at night. Other behaviours affect our sleep in more subtle ways. Your behaviour can interfere with sleep or promote it. Some may look at these recommendations and think, 'I don't need to do this', or 'These changes are too difficult to try, I'll just read on.' These changes are not too difficult; use the exercise to become more determined, and get started!

6

Overcoming worry and anxiety

In this chapter you will learn:
- *about fear and anxiety*
- *how to overcome the fear of insomnia*
- *about the interplay between thoughts, feelings and behaviours*
- *how to control your mind.*

> *There is a time for many words, and there is also a time for sleep*
>
> Homer

Fear and anxiety

Insomnia often leads to anxiety, and with sleeplessness comes a fear of its consequences. Anxiety often leads to insomnia. When half the night is spent worrying about the difficulties in our lives, sleep is stolen from us.

In this chapter, we are going to equip you with the tools required to overcome worry and anxiety. Whether you have come to fear bedtime and the lack of sleep it brings, or whether your mind races with worry as soon as your head hits the pillow, resolving these difficulties will count towards overcoming your insomnia. With NLP techniques, worry-filled sleepless nights can become a thing of the past.

Fear is an experience we have in response to danger. If a person walks down a dark street at night, and they hear fast approaching footsteps, that person would probably be fearful. It would be a rational response to the danger of being robbed or hurt.

Anxiety is also a sense of fear, except the danger isn't real, it is perceived. So if a person walks down a dark street at night and there are no footsteps, to feel fearful at that point would not be rational. There is no danger present. That is anxiety, and it is created in the mind. On some level, they might tell themselves that they are in danger. They are not in danger. It is just a dark street.

Fear of insomnia

So anxiety is a sense of fear where the danger is imagined, rather than real. With insomnia, the danger in question is the danger of tiredness, frustration or emotional upset. If a person experiences many sleepless nights, they will come to anticipate more sleepless nights. Their anticipation will be anxious in nature; worrying about the frustrating experience of lying awake for hours on end.

Once established, a fear of sleepless nights then makes sleepless nights more likely. The reasons for this are two fold. One, anxious states make it difficult to sleep. Two, fearful beliefs are self-fulfilling; our minds are incredibly good at turning our beliefs into reality.

Insight – in the dead of night

Anxieties relating to insomnia can get out of hand: 'What if I lose my job?', 'What if I go insane?', 'What if this kills me?' People do not die from insomnia. Accidents can happen more frequently, but for the most part people tend to cope very well. Insomnia is not going to rob you of your sanity. You might be more emotional, perhaps grumpier than usual, but not insane. And, unless your job involves very repetitive and monotonous work, or incredibly complex work, most job-related impairment will be limited and go unnoticed.

Of course, in the dead of night, with several hours of restless stirring behind you, it is unlikely that you would see it that way. Anxiety is an irrational experience, but a powerful one. When we are in anxious states, our thoughts tend to get stuck in a loop. It is difficult to see sense when you have to be up early the next morning, and particularly when this happens again, and again, and again.

NLP is particularly effective for dealing with anxiety. In this chapter we will guide you through several exercises designed to help. First, we will learn about an exercise that removes phobias, including a phobia of insomnia. This would be an excellent exercise to add to your evening routine. From there, we will look at specific exercises designed to help calm specific anxieties, to be used as and when you need them.

THE FAST PHOBIA CURE (VISUAL KINAESTHETIC DISSOCIATION)

This exercise works very well with irrational fears or phobias. We're going to use it to help with a fear of going to bed and lying awake. It can be tailored to suit most purposes; for example, if you are worried about a meeting the next day.

Have a go

- ▶ This exercise is likely to take around 10 minutes.
- ▶ The best time to use this exercise is when in bed.
- ▶ As you perform the exercise, relax your shoulders and your eyes, and allow yourself to be comfortable.
- ▶ Your concentration will wax and wane a little. After a little practice, you'll be able to remember the steps beforehand so you can perform it fluidly.
- ▶ If you have more than one fear relating to insomnia, use this exercise on the one which creates the strongest feelings of anxiety. You can always focus on other fears when progress is being made.
- ▶ The key to this exercise is repetition.

1   Think about what it is, relating to insomnia, that you are afraid of. It could be an evening of tossing and turning, it could be waking up incredibly tired in the morning. It might be that you'll perform badly at work, lose your job, your house or even your mind. (In our example, we'll focus on a fear of tossing and turning all night.)

2   Make a picture in your mind's eye, if there isn't one already, that represents this fear. Imagine a movie clip of going to bed, tossing and turning, and waking up feeling terrible in the morning. Watch it play in your mind's eye for period of 10 seconds or so.

3   At this point you will be feeling *something*. It could be instantly recognizable as anxiety or worry; it might be more subtle, an alertness, a tingling, a negative feeling in your chest or stomach perhaps.

4   Determine how it is moving through your body. If you need to, gesture with your hand so you get a sense of the movement.

5   When you get a sense of how the feeling is moving, imagine you can reach into the feeling, and reverse it so it moves in the opposite direction (see Chapter 3 for more information

on this). Use your imagination to reach into the feeling, and start to brush it backwards, gently. It helps to tie this into your breathing. Experiment with this, often pushing feelings backwards works best on the out-breath.

6 Push the feeling backwards more and more, so it all starts to spin in the opposite direction. If the feeling was wide, practise making it narrower. If it had a texture, imagine that texture becoming smoother. Many people report that, when a feeling goes backwards, it becomes the opposite feeling. So, anxiety becomes calm. For some people the feeling simply lessens, which is also beneficial.

7 While continuing to spin the feeling backwards, take the frightening mental image which caused this anxiety and change it so it is a) black-and-white; b) dissociated, meaning you can see yourself in the picture; c) small and quite distant in your mind's eye. Note: the image may have disappeared as you focused on the feelings, in which case bring it back and then change it. *Make it look like you're watching the image on a CCTV camera.* Take away any sounds.

8 Imagine you have a remote control for this screen in your mind. In this new mode (black-and-white, small, dissociated and distant – the CCTV view) play it forwards, so you get the gist of what scares you about this mental movie, and then play it backwards, so the mental movie reverses back to the beginning. This will look quite strange, and it will take a few goes to get the order right.

9 Imagine you're playing a tape of this fear forwards, and then backwards. Sometimes the image will flare up into colour and seem to pull you back in. That is quite normal, so simply relax, and do your best to put the mental movie back to the CCTV view: small, black-and-white, distant and dissociated.

10 Now, concentrate on playing the scary mental movie forwards and backwards again, while spinning any negative feelings backwards at the same time. This step will take a little practice.

11 While playing the mental movie forwards and backwards, aim to spin the negative feelings you felt backwards as well. Sometimes they'll ebb away, in which case try to bring them back and have them spin backwards again.

12 Continue this exercise and allow it to become absorbing. While you do, make a conscious effort to relax your eyes, relax your shoulders, and slow your breathing down.

13 After a while, your concentration will wane. When it does, return your focus to the exercise and keep going. When you've learned the steps, the whole exercise should take around 5–10 minutes.

14 Expect your mind to wander as you relax more and more. From there, many people will actually drift off to sleep naturally. See how it works for you.

In essence, this exercise is really simple:

▶ Picture something you fear in your mind's eye and turn it into a movie.
▶ Take any negative feelings you feel at that point and spin them backwards.
▶ Turn the movie into something that looks like it's being filmed on a CCTV camera (small, black-and-white, silent, distant, and dissociated, so you see yourself in the picture).
▶ Play that movie forwards and backwards repeatedly, while continuing to spin the feelings backwards.
▶ Let yourself relax more and more.
▶ Continue for 10 minutes or so.

If you do this for 10 minutes each night in bed, within a few days or so your fear of insomnia will be much less. You're taking the sting out of the negative thoughts that produce anxiety, and you're teaching your body to create new feelings in response to those thoughts. This exercise is incredibly thorough and very powerful.

Practise with this exercise so it works well for you. The more you use it, the more effective it will be.

Insight – NLP is action

If you picture something in your mind's eye so that it is bright, colourful, vivid and realistic, then you'll probably feel strong feelings as a result. If you picture something in your mind's eye so that it's dim, fuzzy, black-and-white, and so you can see yourself in the picture, your body will create much weaker feelings. This has been known for some time. Expensive food packaging is beautifully photographed and brightly coloured, whereas the basic range tends to be packed in simple black-and-white. Out of the two, which seems the most appealing?

Therapists are not the only people to use Neuro-linguistic Programming to change the way you think.

Thoughts, feelings and behaviours

Our thoughts, feelings and behaviours interact, modifying each other. This interaction is the essence of being human, even if we are often not particularly conscious of it. Found within this dynamic interplay are our hopes, our fears and chances of success in life.

Let's take a look at how this affects insomnia. Imagine you are trying to get to sleep with a mind full of anxious thoughts. What effect do these thoughts have on your feelings? Will you be relaxed and ready to sleep, or anxious and unable to drift off? As your prior experiences will no doubt tell you, anxiety is invariably followed by sleeplessness. When you manage to quieten down your mind, sleep then comes easily.

With our thoughts, feelings and behaviours interacting in this way, we can easily become trapped by negative thinking. Thoughts that focus on fatigue will amplify that fatigue, leaving you feeling worse than you needed to. At that point, not all of your fatigue is due to the physiological effects of sleeplessness; some of it is psychological in origin, and therefore avoidable.

It doesn't have to be this way.

Controlling your mind

So if our thoughts, feelings and behaviours are in a state of perpetual interaction, by changing your thoughts, you change this interaction: your emotions and behaviours will reflect your new state of mind. Let's take a look at some exercises that will help you wrestle control of your mind.

THINK FLEXIBLY

Frequently, these exercises will work wonders when you just can't seem to switch off. However, remember the rule we established in Chapter 4? Use your bedroom only for sleeping, reading this book or having sex. Worrying in bed is one of the worst activities you can do. It promotes sleeplessness and rarely solves anything. Getting up after 20 minutes and relaxing for a while usually goes some way towards calming your mind down.

There will be occasions, however, when getting out of bed still leaves your mind in overdrive. Perhaps you are distressed by your sleeplessness, worrying about the consequences of it or anxious about some specific problem you're facing. Here are several exercises designed to help you in such situations.

What we can say for certain is worrying about insomnia only makes it worse. The stress, the anxiety, the doom-laden predictions, how bad we'll feel in the morning. If we look at it rationally, although insomnia is deeply unpleasant, much of the frustration you're feeling is being generated by the way you are looking at it. Let's look at it in a different way.

Imagine a person who absolutely must have £20 on their person at all times. This isn't a matter of preference, it is a matter of urgent importance. If that person were to open their wallet or purse, and find only £10, how would they react? There would be fear, stress and an urgent dash to the cash machine. Fearful, disruptive behaviour based on an idea. They would think, 'I absolutely must have £20 at all times. I must never lose it!' It sounds like a life of stress and misery.

Let's imagine a different person in the same situation. This person prefers to have £20 on their person at all times. It is not an absolute must, just a personal preference. This person opens their purse and also finds only £10. Their reaction? 'I must remember to draw out another £10 later.' Will there be stress or anxiety? Not so much. Instead, they would think, 'I wonder where that £10 went', and carry on with whatever they are doing.

What is the key difference between these two scenarios? Flexibility. In the first example, there is no flexibility, only a hard and fast rule as to what must be. In the second example, a preference is expressed, but it is not a matter of life and death. The person in the second example will live a far happier life than the person in the first. Trying to dictate hard and fast rules gets us nowhere; life does not work like that.

If you feel anxious about your difficulties with insomnia, there has to be some inflexibility in your thinking. You might think, 'But you don't understand! Insomnia is horrible and I'll feel terrible in the morning!' We can agree that insomnia is an unpleasant experience, and we're working together to overcome it. Your insomnia will ease tremendously if you accept it, rather than fight against it. You have a preference, which is to sleep more, but you are treating it more like a demand. And the one thing you cannot demand of yourself is sleep. Accepting that reality will make your recovery much, much easier.

Have a go

▶ This exercise takes moments, and should be used as and when you need it.

▶ It's very straightforward, and over a period of a couple of weeks, it will create a greater flexibility in your thinking.

1 Whenever you think thoughts along the lines of 'This must happen', 'This must not happen', 'I must do this', 'I must not do that' and similar, replace the 'must' with 'prefer'; these thoughts reflect a more realistic view of life.

2 State the new thought, in your mind, in a calm voice. As you do so, relax your shoulders, and look at things more rationally.

Straightforward, as you can see. What types of thought are problematic in their inflexibility? Here are some examples:

▶ I must get to sleep.
▶ I must not be awake.
▶ I can't stand this.
▶ I've got to do something to get some sleep.
▶ I'll feel terrible in the morning

If you think thoughts like this, in a calm voice in your mind, replace them with thoughts such as:

▶ I'd prefer to be asleep, but it's all right to be awake. It'll pass.
▶ I'd prefer not to be awake, but I'll survive. I've survived it before.
▶ I'd prefer not to have to put up with this, but I'll cope. I've coped before.
▶ I'd prefer it if I could sleep, but for now I'll just relax and read this book.
▶ I'd prefer not to feel terrible in the morning, but if I'm tired I'll still manage.

This simple shift from the inflexible to the flexible will make a significant difference to your anxiety. When coping with difficult times, and insomnia *can* be difficult, having a flexible approach will help. You will put yourself under a lot less stress, and therefore sleep more easily.

Sometimes these difficult thoughts don't come in words, they come in pictures. As humans, we tend to think in both. Accompanying vocalized thoughts such as 'I must get to sleep' there may be unpleasant images in your mind's eye. These images might be moving, or still. They might be in full colour and *associated* (as if you were there) or perhaps they'll be dimmer, black-and-white and seen more from a distance. Troubling visual thoughts contribute massively to insomnia. So, let's go through a specific exercise to deal with them.

CALM VISUAL THOUGHTS

Have a go

▶ This exercise takes up to one minute, and should be used as and when you need it.

▶ It is very straightforward. Over a period of a couple of weeks, you will experience fewer and fewer troubling visual thoughts.

1 When you have a troubling visual thought to do with insomnia, perhaps an image of *tossing and turning,* or *looking like death* in the morning, first make the image look like it is being filmed on a CCTV camera: small, black-and-white, so you can see yourself in the picture, and far away.

2 Then, imagine you have a remote control for this screen in your mind. Make the image smaller and smaller, until it becomes the size of a postage stamp.

3 Sometimes, particularly at the start of this process, the image might try to spring back into a full-size colour image. If this happens, then shrink it back down again, and return it to the black-and-white, CCTV mode.

4 When you have the image as a postage stamp-sized image in your mind, tell yourself, 'It's just a stupid thought.'

Combining these two exercises weakens the strength of verbal and visual. Anxiety around insomnia and sleeplessness will reduce greatly, especially with repeated use. These exercises are very effective if you feel troubled about getting up in the early hours (anxiety based on a belief that you *must* be in bed trying to get to sleep). The image to *squash* would be you being in bed, trying to get to sleep, and the words to use would be, 'Even though I'd prefer to be asleep, I'll calm down, relax and I'll be fine.' Something like this.

These exercises combined can also help you to cope with other anxiety-provoking situations. Spend a little time *checking-in* with the images and words which flash through your mind, particularly if you feel anxious. Using these two exercises can help.

DEAL WITH WORRYING SITUATIONS

Relaxation serves as an excellent antidote to worry. Taking a brisk walk or a warm shower (cooling, if you have problems with overheating at night) are excellent ways of clearing your mind. Some people swear by a journal where they record their thoughts and their problems. This can certainly help. If you struggle with day-to-day worries that keep you up at night, these three activities come highly recommended.

Sometimes, though, a warm shower or a brisk walk isn't enough and you need to go a step further. The following exercise is an excellent addition to your toolbox.

Have a go

- ▶ This exercise can take anything from 5 to 25 minutes.
- ▶ You will need a pen and paper. It uses a combination of CBT (Cognitive Behavioural Therapy) and NLP, and is very effective.

1 On a sheet of paper, write down the problem that you cannot stop thinking about. Make your description thorough.
2 Underneath, write the next action or actions you can take to address the situation:
   a If you can resolve it outright, make a note of each action you will need to take.
   b If there are actions you can take that will go some way to resolving the situation, write those down.
   c If you don't know what to do, but can ask somebody, write that down.
   d If there is nothing you can do at the moment, write that down.
   e If you can see it's not such a major situation, write that down.
3 Close your eyes, and picture yourself carrying out the various steps. Use the same submodalities as your *picture of belief*, so the mental movie seems believable. Put in the little details that you can think of.

4 As you visualize this, remind yourself that you're doing everything you can; there's no point feeling bad about it at this point.
5 If there are no steps you can take, then instead picture yourself resolving not to worry, and remind yourself that there is nothing you can do at the moment. There's no point feeling bad about it.
6 When you have completed these steps, place the piece of paper by your bed, folded in half. If at any point you start worrying, re-read the paper, and repeat steps 3 or 4 of this exercise.

This exercise works well in most cases. If you combine the three exercises listed above, you can help yourself to be much more rational, and therefore less anxious, about many things in life. The only thing you can control in life is your reaction to things. If you start with your thoughts, everything else will follow.

So, practise with these exercises. Practise, practise, and practise some more. Use them as frequently as you can, and really get to grips with them. Focus on the array of different fears you might have, starting with the biggest one first. For most people, that will mean either the fear of tossing and turning all night, or the fear of waking up in the morning feeling dreadful. After a week or so, you'll feel a lot more relaxed about going to bed.

Insight – anxiety and the Neurological Levels model

Remember the Neurological Levels Model in Chapter 2? Anxiety is a multi-levelled experience, encompassing our beliefs and values, our skills and knowledge, our thoughts, feelings and behaviour, and our environment. Over time, difficulties with anxiety can even become part of a person's identity.

The exercises in this chapter are mostly focused on the level of thoughts, feelings and behaviour. Overcoming difficulties with anxiety will clear the way for the work we are going to carry out in the next two chapters: learning how to relax (skills and knowledge level) and transforming negative beliefs (beliefs and values level).

In the next chapter we are going to look at relaxation and how it affects sleep. Now would be an excellent time to pause, and practise with the exercises in this chapter (particularly the *fast phobia cure*). In addition to this, review the information in the previous chapters. We learn best by applying knowledge piece by piece. Rather than racing through this book, use the next few days to consolidate what you have learned, and allow the exercises in this chapter to really make a difference.

10 TIPS FOR SUCCESS

1 Insomnia can lead to anxiety, and anxiety often leads to insomnia: either by worrying about the difficulties in our lives or worrying about insomnia itself.

2 Anxiety is a form of fear, where the unpleasant consequences we fear are imagined, rather than real. However, spending many sleepless nights tossing and turning will cause us to fear insomnia even more.

3 People rarely go insane, die or lose their jobs because of insomnia. Even with chronic insomnia, people are resilient and can often cope.

4 When we are in anxious states, our thoughts tend to get stuck in a loop. Getting out of bed can break this cycle.

5 The *fast phobia cure* is a powerful exercise. Irrational fear can be removed quickly and easily using the exercise in this chapter.

6 Our thoughts, feelings and behaviours form a dynamic system; when you think flexibly, your feelings and behaviours will change.

7 Replace inflexible *musts* or *must nots* with the more flexible *prefer*, and anxiety will lessen.

8 Change troubling mental images so they are black-and-white and postage stamp-sized pictures. This will negate the effect they have on the body.

9 Writing down solutions to problems, and visualizing taking the required steps, can help deal with worrying situations.

10 Practising the exercises in this chapter regularly will help you to move beyond fear. Use these exercises for the next seven days or so, and review the previous chapters, before going on to the next.

HOW AM I GETTING ON?

▶ *Have you understood the difference between fear and anxiety? How does this relate to the anxieties that are keeping you up at night?*

▶ *Have you practised* the fast phobia cure *on your fears relating to insomnia?*

▶ *Have you used the exercise to* think flexibly, *rather than inflexibly?*

▶ *Have you practised the exercise to* calm visual thoughts? *What effect does this have?*

▶ *If required, have you practised the exercise to* deal with worrying situations?

Now is a great time to pause and review. Hopefully this book is enjoyable enough for you to want to carry on to the next chapter! Before you do, why not just go over what you've learned so far, and practise. If you consolidate what you have learned so far, you'll build a stronger foundation for what is to come.

7

....

Learning how to relax

In this chapter you will learn:
- *about the difference between tiredness and sleepiness*
- *how your inner voice can help you to sleep*
- *about progressive muscular relaxation*
- *what to do if you can't relax.*

  A ruffled mind makes a restless pillow.

Charlotte Bronte

In Chapters 4 and 5 you were given a list of recommended changes to make, known collectively as *sleep hygiene*. These changes are designed to make your sleeping environment more comfortable, to optimize your body's drive to sleep and to break any negative associations made between your bedroom and insomnia. Now we can turn our attention to creating new, positive associations between your bedroom and sleep.

Conditioned responses are real, and powerful. If you feel a certain way in an environment frequently enough, entering that environment becomes a *cue* to feel that same way in the future. Many people dislike hospitals, for example. Being in hospital often means uncertainty or bad news. As a result, we come to fear or dislike hospitals. Simply dropping off a relative for a routine appointment can create a sense of unease. There is no reason to dislike the hospital at that point but the association has been made so our state changes.

Spending unpleasant, sleepless time in your bedroom has also created a conditioned response, one that is contributing to your insomnia. Instead, we need to create a new response: one of drowsiness. Drowsiness is not the same as tiredness. Over time, your ability to differentiate between these two states may have become scrambled and confused. Insomnia may have left you feeling tired, even exhausted, but feeling tired has not led to more sleep, otherwise there would be no need for this book. Sleep does not follow tiredness, it follows drowsiness.

The difference between tiredness and sleepiness

The difference between feeling tired and feeling drowsy is *relaxation*. When tired you feel heavy, unpleasant, slow... but awake. Drowsiness also feels heavy and slow, but it is a relaxed feeling. You just need to close your eyes, and sleep will surely follow. In this chapter, you are going to learn how to relax and feel drowsy.

To create the positive association we are aiming for, the NLP exercises in this chapter are best carried out before bed, and then while in bed. The other time to practise them, if required, is when you have had to get up and leave your bedroom because you failed to fall asleep within 20 minutes or so. Let's reiterate that advice now.

If you don't fall asleep within 20 minutes of going to bed, get up and relax for 30–60 minutes. Staying in bed, *trying* to get to sleep, is futile and counter-productive. It leads to feelings of frustration and anxiety, which as we have learned only exacerbate insomnia. Aside from the negative conditioning mentioned above, trying and failing to get to sleep is unpleasant. We rarely sleep when we feel unpleasant feelings. Even if you do drift off eventually, your sleep will be light, fractured and not restful. Staying in bed, not sleeping, will still leave you waking up feeling tired. Consider your experiences with insomnia so far, and you will know this to be true.

Insight – resting in bed doesn't work

There is a common misconception that, even if a person isn't sleeping, there is some benefit in lying awake and getting some rest. Recovery does not work in this way. If you're in bed, resting, this will not contribute to feeling better in the morning. Instead, you are just conditioning yourself to struggle with sleep in future. If, after 20 minutes or so, you have not fallen asleep, then it is time to get up and do something relaxing instead.

You might think, 'But I'll feel terrible in the morning!' It is true that you will feel tired the next day if you do not get to sleep until 3 a.m. Beating insomnia is a process; if you only ever fall asleep in bed, then you are educating your body to associate going to bed with falling asleep. This can only be a good thing.

The final point to note, with the relaxation exercises we are going to look at, is that they are designed to bring about deeper sleep. High-quality, deep sleep is our goal. Just six hours of deep, restful sleep is preferable to eight hours of light, fractured sleep. These relaxation exercises take just a little practice. You can't force yourself to relax, so they need to be done slowly. Test out each one, and practise. Experiment. Often these things work best if you apply a little variety.

Do you have an inner monologue? Most of us do. As we wend our way through life, we tend to chatter away to ourselves in our minds. Thoughts, ideas, conclusions, judgements, a running commentary on the day's events; we comment on these things all of the time. This inner monologue is perfectly normal and it can be very difficult to stop.

Let's imagine you are trying to sleep. Tossing and turning, and growing ever more frustrated. Then imagine that somebody is there with you. And this person keeps saying, 'This is taking ages! You'll never get to sleep tonight. You'll feel terrible in the morning... And you've got lots to do tomorrow.' How long before you asked them to leave? There would be choice words, to say the least.

Do you recognize these thoughts as things you have said to yourself in the dead of night? Your inner voice, commentating on your sleeplessness, can make matters much worse. It is a typical problem that is easy to change. There is an excellent NLP technique we can use that will take less than a minute to learn.

Without speaking out loud, can you recite the first few letters of the alphabet in your mind? Good. Now, can you count from one to five? This is your inner voice speaking! Sometimes you will be very aware of it, and sometimes not. It is with this inner voice that we think many of our thoughts.

MAKE YOUR INNER VOICE SLEEPY

Have a go
- ▶ This exercise will take around 1 minute, and for some people it can make *all* of the difference.
- ▶ The key with this exercise is to use it repeatedly.
- ▶ Use it for a couple of minutes before going to bed, and also while in bed.

1 Think about some of the negative things you say to yourself, either before going to sleep, or while trying to sleep. Comments such as, *'I'll never sleep tonight,* or, *'Why can't I get to sleep! I really need to get up in the morning.'*

2 As you run these thoughts through your mind, do they seem to come from the left or the right? From towards the front of your head or the back? Perhaps it sounds like they're outside coming towards you? If so, from which direction? Try repeating a few more negative thoughts about sleep, and determine their location in *your mind's ear.*

3 Now, repeat these same negative thoughts, but imagine they are coming from outside of your window. Think about how that would sound, and make them quieter, more distant.

4 What tone of voice are these thoughts spoken with? Relaxed or happy? Frustrated, angry or resigned?

5 Now, repeat these same negative thoughts, word for word, but use a really content, sleepy voice, like a slow old man or woman settling down for the night.

6 Really slow the thoughts down now, and make them more hushed, more distant, more quiet and calm. Imagine a mother quietly soothing her child to sleep; use that tone of voice with these thoughts and make them sound very, very drowsy.

Ask yourself this question: who is in control here, you or the voice? These are just thoughts in your mind, thoughts that you can control. NLP is an excellent tool for reprogramming our minds to think differently. Thoughts affect our feelings and our behaviours. If you change your thoughts in this way, you'll be amazed at how quickly you feel drowsy.

The best time to start using this exercise is just before you go to bed. Use this sleepy, drowsy voice to think with as you get ready for bed, and keep using it once in bed. It works particularly well with the exercise to *think flexibly* (see Chapter 6) and in conjunction with the rest of the exercises in this chapter.

Insight – develop your sleepy voice

Imagine you've just gone to bed, feeling relaxed and sleepy. And then you think to yourself, *'RIGHT! LET'S GO TO SLEEP! GO TO SLEEP! GO TO SLEEP!'*

It doesn't sound particularly relaxing! Richard Bandler, the co-creator of NLP, likes to mention insomniacs who shout at themselves with their minds. Is your inner voice loud or relaxing?

For some people, overcoming insomnia is simply a case of learning to relax their vocalized and visual thoughts. If you make vocalized thoughts sleepy, and visual images dull and sedate, sleep is much more likely to happen. The exercise to *make your inner voice sleepy* is so simple, but don't let that simplicity mislead you. This is a powerful technique that can really make a difference.

Relaxation

Remember the difference between tiredness and drowsiness? For many people it is relaxation. This exercise is often used by hypnotherapists to promote relaxation in people (this is not a hypnosis exercise, however). Psychologists and psychotherapists will also use this exercise with people because it is simple and effective.

PROGRESSIVE MUSCULAR RELAXATION

Have a go

- ▶ This exercise is likely to take around 10 minutes.
- ▶ Your concentration will wax and wane, and that is to be expected.
- ▶ It is best to use this exercise only while in bed, particularly if you haven't fallen asleep within 10 minutes or so.
- ▶ After a little practice, you'll be able to remember the steps beforehand so you can perform it fluidly.
- ▶ ONLY use this exercise in a place where it safe to relax completely with your eyes closed.

1 First, slow your breathing right down. Consciously focus on your eyelids, and allow them to close and relax. Imagine them becoming heavy, so even if you were to try to open them, it feels like they are too heavy to do so.

2 Focus on your shoulders, make sure they are not tense and hunched, but rather loose and relaxed. Give them a little shake, if you need to.

3 Now, focus on your scalp, and let it gently relax. Using your best *drowsy inner voice*, say to yourself, 'Now I relax my scalp. My scalp is becoming soft... and more relaxed... and let go...'

4 Now, focus on your forehead, and let it gently relax. Using your best *drowsy inner voice*, say to yourself, 'Now I relax my forehead. My forehead is becoming soft... and more relaxed... and let go...'

5 Now, focus on your eyelids, and let them gently relax. Using your best *drowsy inner voice*, say to yourself, 'Now I relax my eyelids. My eyelids are becoming soft... and more relaxed... and let go...'

6 Now, focus on your face, and let it gently relax. Using your best *drowsy inner voice*, say to yourself, 'Now I relax my face. My face is becoming soft... and more relaxed... and let go...'

7 Now, focus on your jaw, and let it gently relax. Using your best *drowsy inner voice*, say to yourself, 'Now I relax my jaw. My jaw is becoming soft... and more relaxed... and let go...'

8 Now, focus on the back of your neck, and let it gently relax. Using your best *drowsy inner voice*, say to yourself, 'Now I relax the back of my neck. The back of my neck is becoming soft... and more relaxed... and let go...'

9 Now, focus on your shoulders, and let them gently relax. Using your best *drowsy inner voice*, say to yourself, 'Now I relax my shoulders. My shoulders are becoming soft... and more relaxed... and let go...'

10 Now, focus on your upper arms, and let them gently relax. Using your best *drowsy inner voice*, say to yourself, 'Now I relax my upper arms. My upper arms are becoming soft... and more relaxed... and let go...'

11 Now, focus on your lower arms, and let them gently relax. Using your best *drowsy inner voice*, say to yourself, 'Now I relax my lower arms. My lower arms are becoming soft... and more relaxed... and let go...'

12 Now, focus on your hands, and let them gently relax. Using your best *drowsy inner voice*, say to yourself, 'Now I relax my hands. My hands are becoming soft... and more relaxed... and let go...'

13 Now, focus on your chest muscles, and let them gently relax. Using your best *drowsy inner voice*, say to yourself, 'Now I relax my chest. My chest is becoming soft... and more relaxed... and let go...'

14 Now, focus on your upper back, and let it gently relax. Using your best *drowsy inner voice*, say to yourself, 'Now I relax my upper back. My upper back is becoming soft... and more relaxed... and let go...'

15 Now, focus on your lower back, and let it gently relax. Using your best *drowsy inner voice*, say to yourself, 'Now I relax my lower back. My lower back is becoming soft... and more relaxed... and let go...'

16 Now, focus on your stomach muscles, and let them gently relax. Using your best *drowsy inner voice*, say to yourself, 'Now I relax my stomach. My stomach is becoming soft... and more relaxed... and let go...'

17 Now, focus on your thigh muscles, and let them gently relax. Using your best *drowsy inner voice*, say to yourself, 'Now I relax my thighs. My thighs are becoming soft... and more relaxed... and let go...'

18 Now, focus on your calves, and let them gently relax. Using your best *drowsy inner voice*, say to yourself, 'Now I relax my calves. My calves are becoming soft... and more relaxed... and let go...'

19 Now, focus on your feet, and let them gently relax. Using your best *drowsy inner voice*, say to yourself, 'Now I relax my feet. My feet are becoming soft... and more relaxed... and let go...'

20 Now, focus on your mind, and the fuzzy space behind your eyelids, and imagine that your mind is become more and more fuzzy, and relaxed. Using your best *drowsy inner voice*, say to yourself, 'Now I relax my mind. My mind is becoming soft... and more relaxed... and let go...'

Repeat Step 20, really slowly, for the next few minutes, and when you say to yourself, 'and let go...' let yourself relax even more. Use this exercise only when it is safe to relax completely. Never use this exercise if driving or operating machinery, for example.

The trick to this exercise is to do it slowly. Rather than racing through it, trying to relax, you have to be gentle, take your time, and let it happen. You cannot force yourself to relax; the very idea doesn't make sense. Relaxation happens when you stop trying, so instead just let it go. Although there are 20 steps in this exercise, ultimately it is the same, slow, soporific affirmation, to *relax a part of your body, and to let go.*

Have a go

▶ This exercise is likely to take 5–10 minutes.
▶ Your concentration will wax and wane during this exercise, and that is a good sign.
▶ The best time to use this exercise is in bed.
▶ As you perform the exercise, relax your shoulders, your eyes, and allow yourself to be comfortable.
▶ After a little practice, you'll be able to remember the steps beforehand so you can perform it fluidly.
▶ Only use this exercise in a place where it safe to relax completely with your eyes closed.

1 Consciously focus on your eyelids, and allow them to relax. Imagine them becoming heavy, so even if you were to try to open them, it feels like they are too heavy to do so.
2 Focus on your shoulders, and make sure they are not tense and hunched, but rather loose and relaxed. Give them a little shake, if you need to.
3 Remember a time when you felt very drowsy. It could be a time before your insomnia started, or it could be a time when you managed to sleep well recently.
4 As you recall the time when you were very drowsy, place yourself into the memory as if it were happening now. Relax into it, and allow yourself to believe that it is happening now. It's like when you watch a film: you suspend disbelief. Imagine that you're there, feeling heavy, drowsy, and increasingly comfortable.
5 Take whichever drowsy feelings you feel, and imagine you can gently spread them around your body. This is like the *spinning feelings* exercise we practised in Chapter 3. This time, imagine you're spreading feelings around slowly, comfortably and in a relaxed way.
6 Remember how it feels when you want to yawn? Focus on how that feels and, even if you have to give the process a little nudge to begin with, try a yawn now. After a moment or two, often this becomes a real yawn.

Again, the trick to making this exercise work is to do it slowly. If you have any thoughts running through your mind, make them hushed and slow. As you move feelings around your body, do that slowly, and gently, like syrup almost. Remember that feeling of being engrossed in a film? Approach this exercise with the same mentality. You're aiming for it to absorb your imagination.

Combine this exercise with the exercise to *make your inner voice sleepy* described earlier, for best effect.

GUIDED IMAGERY

Guided imagery is another form of visualization that can help when you need to sleep. To some extent, our body responds to the imagined as if it were real. Let's try an experiment. Now, if you were to imagine a fresh, bright yellow lemon – juicy, the smell of it, the zest... Imagine you're slicing into it, cutting the lemon in half. The flesh is glistening. You're almost able to taste the zest already. Imagine, now, taking the lemon in your hand, and smelling the freshness of it. The sharpness of it. And then biting into it... Your mouth watering as you taste fresh lemon juice...

There's a good chance your mouth is watering? This is the power of your imagination. Using guided imagery to aid sleep works on the same principle.

Have a go

▶ This exercise is likely to take around 5 minutes.

▶ Your concentration will wax and wane during this exercise, and that is a good sign.

▶ The best time to use this exercise is after the *progressive muscular relaxation* exercise above.

- ▶ After a little practice, you'll be able to remember the steps beforehand so you can perform it fluidly.
- ▶ Only use this exercise when it safe to relax completely with your eyes closed.

1 In a moment close your eyes, and imagine you're walking slowly along a path, through a light forest. Utilize your internal senses. Make the images bright and clear, so it feels like you are in that space.
2 Imagine the sounds of birds. Feel the cool air on your skin. Smell the freshness of the forest... a forest that you might remember from when you were young...
3 Imagine slowly walking down this forest path, until you find a bench, bathed in gentle sunlight. Warming your skin, and helping you to relax...

Spend 5 minutes or so imagining this scene. Engage all of your senses. Slow down your breathing. Relax your eyelids, and your shoulders. Suspend your disbelief so that you can imagine you are there... Let's try that now.

***

Welcome back! How did that feel? There's a good chance that it took you a while to get into it, and that your mind wandered. With practice, using this type of imagery can really aid sleep. The very best time to do this is in bed, after the *progressive muscular relaxation* exercise. Relaxing scenes work best, but scenes that mean something to you will be the most effective. Draw on your imagination and see where it takes you.

PUTTING THIS TOGETHER

Your sleeping environment should now be much more comfortable and conducive to sleep, and your daily routine more focused on promoting sleep, rather than detracting from it. Old fears and negative conditioning are being dismantled. From this point forward, a much healthier, positive association between your bedroom and sleep will be formed. Being strict with yourself regarding the list of what to do (and what not to do) in your bedroom will continue to reinforce this process.

Now it is time to learn to relax. Relaxation plays a vital role in transforming fatigue into sleepiness. In the next chapter, we will remove any negative beliefs that are interfering with your recovery from insomnia. Before we get to that, it would make sense to really practise with the exercises in this chapter. For many, they will make all the difference, which leads us on to our final recommendation for now.

What to do if you cannot relax

If, having followed all of the recommendations in this book so far, you don't fall asleep after 20 minutes or so, and you just know you are not going to sleep at any point soon, the best thing to do is *get up!* Yes, we've discussed this before but it is a point worth repeating! Let's take a look at the pros and cons.

Advantages of getting out of bed if you cannot sleep:

▶ You avoid the frustration, anxiety and tension of lying in bed, awake.
▶ You avoid strengthening the negative conditioning that is contributing to your insomnia.
▶ You do strengthen, however, the understanding that your bedroom is for sleep only.
▶ Although you are tired, you are not yet sleepy. It is far better for your mental health to accept that fact, rather than ignoring it.
▶ You will have extra time to read this book and practise the exercises.

Disadvantages of getting out of bed if you cannot sleep:

▶ You may have to get dressed and potentially disturb someone.
▶ You will be as tired as you would have been if you'd stayed in bed.

Sometimes people feel that getting up is admitting defeat. In fact, getting up teaches your body to sleep more easily in future; it is not defeat, but progress. If you use the various relaxation exercises in this chapter and still don't feel sleepy, then you have tried enough for now. Get up, do something else instead, and then after 30–60 minutes or so, try again.

The exercises in this chapter, and the *fast phobia cure* exercise in Chapter 6, are good to practise at such times. As you practise these exercises, remember to ensure that your eyelids are relaxed, your shoulders are relaxed, and that you're sitting comfortably. With practice, these exercises become easier and more effective.

Sometimes you might not feel like practising these exercises (and fair enough). We all need a break sometimes. At such times, try to avoid activities that depend on a screen, such as watching TV or surfing the internet. Some people swear that reading fiction helps them sleep, whereas others find that it keeps them awake. Experiment and find out if this helps or hinders your efforts. Reading non-fiction work should be fine. Caffeinated drinks should obviously be avoided.

Remember, the nature of change is rarely a straight line from A to B. Usually there will be improvements, followed by setbacks, followed by further improvements, and so on. Sometimes things bumble along a bit, and then click into place. Stick with the exercises, and be strict with yourself when it comes to following the recommendations and practising the exercises. Change does happen; people do reconnect with their natural ability to sleep.

In the next chapter, we will look at those beliefs that can get in the way.

10 TIPS FOR SUCCESS

1 Conditioned responses are real and powerful; the recommendations we have put in place so far are designed to undo those responses, so we can programme better ones.

2 Feeling tired and feeling sleepy are not the same thing. Feeling sleepy is likely to lead to sleep. Feeling tired will not. The difference between the two, in most cases, is relaxation.

3 Using relaxation exercises in bed will condition you to associate your bedroom with relaxation, and eventually sleep.

4 If you don't fall asleep within 20 minutes of getting into bed, simply get up and practise some of the exercises in this book.

5 Your inner voice chatters away all of the time, which is unhelpful when trying to sleep. With just a little practice, you can make your inner voice sound tired and sleepy.

6 Progressive muscular relaxation involves systematically relaxing each part of your body, while using your sleepy inner voice to affirm and reinforce that relaxation. Hypnotherapists sometimes use this method to help people relax, and it is well worth practising.

7 You can teach yourself to feel drowsy by remembering what it feels like to be in a sleepy state. Gently amplify those feelings using the NLP spinning techniques we practised in Chapter 3.

8 Guided imagery is sleep-inducing, especially after using the *progressive muscular relaxation* exercise.

9 Lying in bed, trying to get to sleep, will only make matters worse. You will end up frustrated, perhaps anxious, and negative conditioning will be reinforced.

10 Remember: if you don't fall asleep within 20 minutes of trying, then get up and practise some of the exercises in this chapter. (A point *so important*, it is worth stating twice!)

HOW AM I GETTING ON?

▶ *Have you understood the difference between feeling tired and feeling sleepy?*

▶ *Have you practised making your inner voice sound slow, sleepy and relaxed?*

▶ *Have you practised the* progressive muscular relaxation *exercise while in bed?*

▶ *Have you practised with the exercise to* feel drowsy at bedtime?

▶ *Have you practised with* guided imagery? *What visualization do you find most relaxing?*

▶ *Have you got out of bed, if required, because you did not fall asleep within 20 minutes or so?*

If you can answer yes to the questions above, there is a good chance that you are already getting more sleep. Well done for being so thorough. You're well on the way to recovery.

If you cannot answer yes to all of the questions above, now would be an excellent time to pause, reflect and follow the suggestions and recommendations in this chapter carefully. The programme you are following is straightforward, but there is a lot to get your head around, and it can take time to put it all in place. Persevere, and you will progress. In the next chapter, we'll go through some very useful work based around negative, limiting beliefs around insomnia.

8

Transforming negative beliefs

In this chapter you will learn:
- *about the limiting nature of belief*
- *about deletions, generalizations and distortions*
- *about some typical sleep myths*
- *how to change your limiting beliefs.*

> *To succeed, we must first believe that we can.*
>
> Michael Korda

In the previous chapter we went through an array of exercises designed to promote relaxation and sleepiness. As we've already learned, there is a difference between feeling tired and feeling sleepy. These exercises, coupled with the recommendations made earlier in this book, will go a long way to helping you beat insomnia.

Relaxation is important, but there are many different factors that can cause sleeplessness. In this chapter, we are going to focus on the negative beliefs that often get in the way of sleep. Insomnia has a psychological dimension: *sleep myths*, that hold us back.

The effect of belief on consciousness

In Chapter 3 we touched on the nature of belief. Beliefs inform our experience of reality. They are learned conclusions: ideas that we hold with conviction. People will argue endlessly over sport, politics or religion, because people believe different things, and their beliefs are real to them. For some, it is incomprehensible that others might believe something different.

You will have acquired beliefs about sleep in general, and about your sleep in particular. Your beliefs about sleep guide you, shaping your perceptions of how things should be or shouldn't be, and what to expect. Your beliefs seem real to you, but how do you know that your beliefs are accurate or true?

For example, do you feel that eight hours' sleep is the right amount of sleep for you? Can you pinpoint the origin of this belief? Unless you have filled out a sleep diary for many years documenting the evidence, is your belief supported by fact or is it just an idea, something you hold to be true without knowing why?

As people, we often learn from others. Much of what we learn this way helpfully guides us: the conventional wisdom. The problem with conventional wisdom is that it is often superseded by subsequent academic consensus. Also, conventional wisdom can become distorted as it is passed from person to person. We often hold beliefs that we simply don't understand.

Insight – the nature of belief

I recently caught up with an old friend at a wedding. In the news that day was a story about water being found on Mars. We were discussing this, and he mentioned that Mars was the third planet in the solar system. I attempted to correct him: Earth is the third planet, and Mars is the fourth. He became increasingly upset and belligerent. At school, somehow, he'd acquired the belief that Mars was the third planet, and didn't take kindly to being told otherwise! After a while, I gave up. He didn't want to listen.

This demonstrates the nature of belief. Sometimes we blindly defend them, no matter how irrational they might seem to others. After a while my friend knew he was mistaken, deep down, but still he remained belligerent. One of the things we really hate, as human beings, is to be wrong. Sometimes we just need to let go of our limiting beliefs, particularly if we want to find lasting change.

Your beliefs about sleep may be contributing to your insomnia. If a belief is a learned conclusion, then there has been a conclusion to the learning. In the example above, my friend was angry that his belief was being challenged, even though his belief was inaccurate. Are your beliefs about sleep accurate or do they limit you in some way?

Let's shed some light on how beliefs can lack nuance and sophistication.

Deletions, generalizations and distortions

DELETIONS

In our thinking, we often delete things. Have you ever written a sentence, only to find a deleted? Apologies! Only to find a *word* deleted? We delete things all the time. As you read this book, are you aware of your big toe? Unlikely: your big toe is (most probably) there, but it is not important to the task of reading, so your brain deletes it from your awareness. If you were to suddenly get cramp in your toe, your brain would *undelete* your awareness of it, via discomfort or pain.

On some level, you might believe that you are a poor sleeper. However, there have been times in your life when you have slept well, even if just once or twice. You might bristle at this assertion, just as my friend bristled when his belief about Mars was challenged. Only with a comprehensive and accurate record of your sleep, dating back to your birth, could you assert your belief is absolutely correct. Without that record, there is no evidence to support the idea that you have never been able to sleep well, even if you believe it is the truth.

Believing that you cannot sleep well contributes to insomnia: a self-fulfilling prophecy. This is a belief of inevitability, and it renders you helpless and hopeless. Here, you are deleting the possibility of learning how to find better sleep. If you believe that you are a poor sleeper, changing this limiting conclusion will help.

GENERALIZATIONS

At school you learned the letters of the alphabet. You can recognize those letters in this text. The letters printed here are not precisely the same as the ones you learned to recognize. Those letters, written on a blackboard or an exercise book, are long gone. This is a type of generalization.

We learn by generalizing, and this can be helpful: imagine if you had to relearn the alphabet every time you wanted to read something. Unfortunately, things can sometimes go wrong. If a little boy is bitten by a dog and is then scared, in pain and upset he might conclude, 'Dogs are scary! They bite and I don't like them.'

With this belief now formed, his fear will generalize to all dogs; even the most decrepit and toothless poodle will frighten him! This generalization is far from useful. Dogs don't always bite and the fear is unnecessary.

You may have had extensive, debilitating periods of insomnia in your life. You might conclude, 'Insomnia is terrible! I'll never be able to sleep properly again.' This generalization is also far from useful. Experiencing insomnia in the past does not mean you always will. Things change, and you can learn to find better sleep. You may not believe that, but your belief is just an idea that you hold with conviction. Only as you draw your last breath would you be able to state truly, 'Yes, I never got the hang of sleeping.' And at that point, you are not likely to care! Until then, your predictions for future sleeplessness are just generalizations that are holding you back.

DISTORTIONS

Imagine an ambitious young man going for a promotion. He doesn't get the job, and angrily concludes, 'My boss doesn't like me!' Perhaps this is true, or perhaps the successful candidate gave a better interview. His conclusion, at that point, is an example of distorted thinking. (It does not matter if he is right: even a stopped clock tells the right time twice per day. He arrived at this conclusion via angry thinking, not reasoned insight.)

Insight – distorted thinking

Imagine that you're out with a group of friends. As you leave to go to the bathroom, they all burst out laughing. You flush with insecurity or anger, as if they're laughing at you. Rationally, you know they've probably just shared a joke. Emotionally, you might feel angry as if the joke was at your expense.

This is an example of distorted thinking. Your reasoning is distorted at that moment; your view of matters has little to do with what is going on in reality. Our thinking about insomnia can be incredibly distorted. Because sleeplessness can be a bit of a mystery sometimes, we are left prone to illogical guesswork rather than reasoned fact.

Tiredness leaves us vulnerable to distorted thinking, and there are many myths and misconceptions surrounding sleep. If you believe you cannot overcome insomnia for any particular reason, that is most likely a distorted thought. You don't know that you cannot overcome your insomnia. It is a guess, and it is holding you back.

Our beliefs regarding sleep frequently lack logic. Have you ever thought to yourself:

▶ I've never slept well.
▶ Other people can sleep better than I can.
▶ Insomnia runs in the family.
▶ I'll never get over my insomnia.
▶ I've always been an insomniac.
▶ I need eight hours' sleep.
▶ Insomnia is killing me!
▶ No matter what I try, it's bound to fail.
▶ My insomnia means I never get enough sleep.
▶ I didn't sleep at all last night.
▶ I didn't sleep at all last night and that means I'll have a terrible day today.
▶ I had no sleep last night and I know I'll have no sleep tonight.
▶ I'm going to lose my job / house / mind / etc. because of this damned insomnia!
▶ I just can't sleep.

Each of these statements contains deletions, generalizations or distortions. All three in some cases. You might recognize some of these statements as your own, but that does not mean that they are accurate or true.

IDENTIFYING DELETIONS, GENERALIZATIONS AND DISTORTIONS

Have a go
Go through the list of statements above and write next to each thought whether you think it is a deletion (D), a generalization (G), a distortion (X), or any combination of the three. It will only take a moment to consider each one. Once you have completed the exercise, see which statements you can identify with, from your own experience, and consider the effect such thoughts have on your sleep.

How did you do? If you identified with a particular statement, perhaps you can now see the limiting effect it is having on your efforts to improve your sleep. Such beliefs form a mental prison; we can free your mind with this simple exercise.

CHANGE LIMITING BELIEFS (BELIEF CHANGE PROCESS)

This exercise transforms limiting beliefs. By changing such beliefs, your insomnia will improve and you will sleep more easily. It is as simple as that.

The exercise to *change limiting beliefs* is best done in three stages. Complete each stage in sequence, and ideally in the same session. The first stage of this exercise is very similar to the *fast phobia cure* in Chapter 6.

Have a go

▶ This first part of the exercise takes anywhere between 10 and 20 minutes.
▶ Choose one limiting belief to work with.
▶ Carry out the exercise once per day for around seven days.
▶ If you're unsure as to which belief to start with, begin with the belief that you'll always struggle to sleep.

1 Close your eyes and make a visual representation of the negative belief you want to change. As an example, you could make a mental movie of going to bed, tossing and turning, getting up, eventually falling asleep but feeling terrible the next day.
2 Take a little time to build up how this mental movie looks; the order in which the story unfolds. Relax. Concentrate, and put in place those details that reflect your belief.
3 Visualize the movie clip as if it were playing on a CCTV screen: elevated camera angle, black-and-white, small screen, and so it is dissociated (you can watch yourself in the picture).
4 Play the movie clip forwards, for around 10–20 seconds or so. Spend a bit of time building up how it looks, so it makes sense to you.
5 Then, take the movie clip and run it backwards; from the end to the beginning. Again, take a little time with it, and work out how it all looks when it plays backwards.
6 Play it forwards and then backwards, two times in total. Take a little time to settle on the order of events and the way it looks. At this point, if your mental movie has sounds, make it silent.
7 Open and close your eyes. Then play it forwards and backwards three times in total.

8 Then, open and close your eyes. Now play it forwards and backwards five times in total.

9 During this process, although you're aiming to keep it small, black-and-white, and dissociated, you might find that your mind wants it to become colourful, large, and pull you into it, as if you were there. This is normal to begin with. It will get much easier to keep it black-and-white as the exercise progresses.

10 Now, play the image repeatedly forwards and backwards five times. Then open and close your eyes.

11 Repeat Step 10 several times. In time, you'll notice that it gets easier to keep it black-and-white, small and dissociated. Keep going. Play it forwards and backwards, in groups of five. After each group of five, open and close your eyes.

12 After a while longer, you'll notice that the movie seems to speed up. This is always a good sign. Keep going still. After around 10 minutes of repetitious playing (forwards and backwards, in groups of five, opening and closing your eyes after each group of five plays), you will start to feel very detached from the movie clip. Keep going.

13 At some point, you'll notice that the person in the movie clip doesn't really look or feel like you, as if you're watching something on TV. At that point, keep repeating Step 10, just for a little while longer.

14 One of three things might happen: (a) the image might just keep disintegrating – if so, try to bring the image back, and keep going; (b) you might start to find it incredibly amusing, and again that's a good sign – keep going; (c) you might start to realize that it's just a limiting belief, and again, that is also a good sign – keep going.

15 Then, put yourself right in the picture, so you imagine you're in the middle of the mental movie. How does that feel? If there is any anxiety, certainty or emotional connection, then repeat Step 10 for a further 5 minutes or so.

16 When you feel emotionally disconnected from the image, we've completed the first phase of our work in this exercise.

The second part of the exercise is very straightforward, and takes around 2 minutes to complete. If required, refer to your answers to the *picture of belief* exercise (Chapter 3). We're going to utilize the submodalities of that visualization now.

118

17 Picture yourself doing the opposite of the belief you've been
    working with. So, in our example, this would be you sleeping
    soundly and waking up refreshed.
18 Make a mental movie of you doing just that; put in place those
    details that prove you're sleeping well; looking sleepy and
    relaxed, getting to sleep quickly and waking up refreshed.
19 Good. So, in a moment, take this mental movie and *snap!* it so
    it takes on all of the qualities present in your *picture of belief*
    (Chapter 3). Make it have exactly the same level of colour,
    brightness, focus and position in your mind's eye. This should
    take around 1 second, maximum.
20 Repeat Step 19 ten times. It will take around 10 seconds to do.
    Open and close your eyes in between each go.
21 Now, repeat Step 19 a further ten times! It is best to be
    thorough with this type of work.

When you have finished this exercise, take a moment or two to look
at the limiting belief more rationally, with a scientific eye, and notice
that it feels different. Within a week or so, limiting beliefs will be
transformed. Use this exercise repeatedly.

Insomnia has a psychological dimension. If you can dispel anxiety in
the short term, and evolve your beliefs to be more rational in the long
term, your mind will help you sleep. That can only be a good thing.

In Chapter 9, we are going to begin troubleshooting the programme
so far. This step is key to your recovery, and we'll go through it
thoroughly next.

10 TIPS FOR SUCCESS

1 Insomnia is complex. There are many factors to consider, including negative, limiting beliefs about sleep.

2 Beliefs inform our experience of reality. They are learned conclusions; ideas that we hold with conviction.

3 Conventional wisdom isn't always accurate. Our beliefs often lack nuance and interfere with our ability to sleep.

4 You may believe that eight hours' sleep is the right amount of sleep for you, but this is just an idea; something you hold to be true without knowing why.

5 We constantly delete things from our awareness. When it comes to your ability to sleep, or the quality of your sleep, you might be deleting information that could improve your experience.

6 We learn by making generalizations: imagine if you had to relearn the alphabet every time you wanted to read something. Sometimes our ability to generalize causes problems. For example, having insomnia in the past does not mean you will suffer with it indefinitely.

7 Our reasoning, when it comes to insomnia, is often distorted. If you believe you cannot overcome insomnia for any reason, that is most likely a distorted thought.

8 By changing limiting beliefs about sleep, your insomnia will improve and you will sleep more easily.

9 The process of changing beliefs is very straightforward. It follows two stages: a) make a visual representation of your belief, and desensitize it via repeated CCTV-style visualization; b) take a visual representation of what you would prefer to believe, and make it look more believable.

10 The exercise to *change limiting beliefs* works best when you do it repeatedly. Managing troubling thoughts in the short term and limiting beliefs in the long term will help you find better sleep.

HOW AM I GETTING ON?

▶ *Have you read and understood the information in this chapter on deletions, generalizations and distortions?*

▶ *Have you looked at the list of typical negative beliefs and decided whether they are deletions, generalizations or distortions (or a combination of the three)?*

▶ *Have you chosen a limiting belief and practised with the belief change process?*

When you can answer yes to the questions above, you have overcome another hurdle between you and good quality sleep. Insomnia has a psychological component, which must not be discounted. We underestimate how profoundly our beliefs govern and shape us.

In the next chapter, we are going to begin troubleshooting the programme so far. This step is key to your recovery, and we'll go through it thoroughly. You do have the innate ability to sleep. Alongside breathing, it is one of the most natural things we do. By now, you might be starting to believe that.

9

Troubleshooting problems with your sleep

In this chapter you will learn:
- *how to use your sleep diary to pinpoint sleep problems*
- *how to overcome specific sleep difficulties*
- *how to put the full programme together.*

> *I will either find a way, or make one.*
>
> Hannibal

In this chapter, we are going to pinpoint any outstanding problems with sleeplessness. We will then start fine-tuning the changes you have made so far, and sleep will continue to improve.

Using your sleep diary to identify trends, patterns and inertia

If you have been following the recommendations carefully, by now you will have accomplished the following:

▶ Made positive changes to your sleeping environment (see Chapter 4), so that it is more comfortable.
▶ Made changes to certain behaviours, such as keeping to a regular rising time, designed to increase your drive to sleep.
▶ Used exercises to help deal with anxious thoughts and feelings.
▶ Used exercises to help you to relax.
▶ Used the exercise to *change limiting beliefs* about sleep.
▶ Filled in your sleep diary for the past 14–21 days or so.

Looking at your sleep diary, what is the overall picture? Has there been an increase in the ease with which you have got to sleep? Has there been an increase in the quality of your sleep? If you have implemented the changes in this book, the answers to these questions should be yes. At the very least, your sleep diary should give you an accurate overview of your sleeping habits.

We are looking for trends, patterns and problem areas:

▶ **Trends** are gradual improvements over the weeks you have been using this book.
▶ **Patterns** are difficulties that keep recurring; for example, finding it difficult to go to sleep on Sunday nights.
▶ **Problem areas** are unsatisfactory situations that are not responding to the changes you have made; for example, little or no improvement in the number of times you're waking up each night.

DECODING YOUR SLEEP DIARY

Have a go

Your sleep diary is vital to this next stage of the programme. Take a look at the various rows of information, and get a handle on what has happened with your sleep in these past few weeks. Spend a good 10–20 minutes going through each row, looking for trends, patterns and problem areas.

Sleep aids and alcohol

Look at the information in this row, do you see any pattern? It could be frequent use of sleep aids or that you turn to such aids at certain times. If you are using sleeping pills regularly, this is a situation that may be worth reviewing with your GP.

Frequently using alcohol to aid the onset of sleep will interfere with the quality of sleep you get. There is more information on alcohol in the troubleshooting guide, below.

Time I went to bed and *Time it took to fall asleep*

Take a look at the *Time I went to bed* and *Time it took to fall asleep* rows. Does the time (that you first attempted to go to bed) vary or is it consistent? Is it later at the weekends? Perhaps there is a different pattern you can recognize?

Did you manage to stick to the rule of not spending more than 20 minutes trying to get to sleep?

Next, take a look at the number of times you tried to get to sleep. This lets us know how easy you found it to get to sleep each night. If you did follow the rule of not spending more than 20 minutes in bed, then there might be occasions where you 'went to bed' several times each night. Again, look for a pattern. Is this worse at the start of the week, the end of the week or at the weekends? Do certain life-events interfere with your ability to fall asleep? Have these figures improved over the past couple of weeks?

Ideally, you will be getting to sleep on the first attempt more frequently as you act on the recommendations we've discussed.

Did I use the NLP exercises from Chapters 5–7?

Did you use the NLP exercises when required? What impact did they have on your ability to fall sleep? Has your ability to fall asleep, or re-fall asleep, improved in the past three weeks?

Did you find that, with practice, the exercises became easier? Perhaps the opposite is true and you grew complacent, not using the exercises as thoroughly as you did at the beginning. Either of these scenarios might be reflected in your ability to fall asleep more easily.

Number of times I awoke during the night

Each night, on average, how many times did you wake up? Has that value changed over the course of the past two to three weeks? Ideally, we want this figure to get lower as the weeks progress. Is that the case?

Length of time spent trying to get back to sleep

If you did wake in the night, how long did it take you to get back to sleep? Did you stick to the 20-minute rule?

Did I use the NLP exercises from Chapters 5–7?

If you did wake during the night, did you try the NLP exercises designed to help you get back to sleep? If so, did they help, and to what extent? Has the efficacy of these exercises improved or declined over the past few weeks?

Final waking time

Reviewing the data for the whole two to three weeks, is there a typical waking time or does it vary? Is there a discernible pattern, such as much later waking times at the weekends, for example?

Time I got out of bed

Take a look at the information in this row, especially in relation to the row above, your *final waking time*. Did you spend more than 20 minutes in bed after waking?

I woke up x minutes earlier than I wanted to (last waking)

Are you finding that you sleep until your ideal waking time, or are you waking up too early? If so, is there a pattern, again considering weekends or typical life-events? Has this figure evolved over the past two to three weeks?

Quality of sleep on a scale of 1–5 (1 = very poor; 5 = excellent)

Reviewing the data here for the past few weeks, what score have you given your sleep? Is it consistent, or does it vary? Is there a pattern? If so, does that pattern correlate with the other rows in your sleep diary? If the score you have given your sleep is consistently bad, have you taken into account any improvements that you are noticing, such as getting to sleep more easily? Spend a little time, and see if you can identify the trends, patterns and problem areas that exist in your sleep diary.

Using your sleep diary to troubleshoot problems

By looking at the data in your sleep diary, we can begin to troubleshoot problems. Insomnia is complicated and idiosyncratic. If you have followed the steps in this book carefully, there is a very good chance that your insomnia is improving. For some, there will still be significant hurdles to overcome. Using the information contained in your sleep diary will help.

Let's go through the problems that might still exist, and come up with some possible solutions.

I AM NOT FILLING IN MY SLEEP DIARY

Being honest, did you managed to fill in your sleep diary consistently? For some, filling in the sleep diary will have been straightforward; for others, there might be gaps, or even nothing at all.

If you've struggled to fill in your sleep diary, consider how that has happened. Has the problem been a practical one, such as not having it to hand, with a pen, by your bed? Have you forgotten to fill it in on some days, and then let it fall by the wayside? Is there a clear, practical reason why you haven't been able to utilize your sleep diary fully? If so, re-read Chapter 1 and ask yourself the question, 'Do I want to tackle this problem, or not?'

It could be that the problem is psychological rather than practical. People often feel reluctant to start something new. There are several factors that might come in to play. You might fear starting with your sleep diary because you fear that you won't persist with it. This might seem irrational, and it is! When we fear that we will fail at something, we often avoid starting it in the first place.

Perhaps you are afraid that, by filling in your sleep diary, you will only record a lack of progress. This is *a fear of failure* in another form. There might be an unconscious resistance to filling in your sleep diary in case you record information that challenges your beliefs about insomnia. Some may worry, '*What if it's something other than insomnia? Then what?*' A thought like this, at the back of your mind, is going to leave you feeling averse to recording your sleeping patterns.

> ### Insight – the importance of your sleep diary
>
> For some people, the idea of filling out a sleep diary can seem like too much hassle: '*Oh, I don't need to do that, I'll just try out some exercises instead.*' On reading this chapter, it should have become clear that a sleep diary is an excellent tool for troubleshooting problems. If you've decided to exempt yourself from completing this small task each day, consider un-exempting yourself!
>
> Filling in your sleep diary takes a minute or two each morning, and provides a rich source of data that will help you immensely.

So, in the case of a psychological factor (or factors) acting as a barrier between you and completing the sleep diary, there are two important steps you can take. Use the *fast phobia cure* (see Chapter 6). Visualize a mental movie of avoiding, or forgetting, to fill in your sleep diary. Repeat the exercise several times, until you start to see the task for what it is. Quick, simple and beneficial.

Once completed, re-read Chapter 1, and complete the exercise to *fill in your sleep diary* in Chapter 3. You'll have a much clearer picture of what you are aiming to achieve.

RELIANCE ON SLEEP MEDICATIONS

Sleep medication, when not used excessively, can be of great benefit to those who struggle with sleep. Especially when used in conjunction with a programme designed to improve sleep, such as this book.

Problems can arise. People with insomnia lose confidence in their ability to sleep. We then look for things that support us, rather than working to regain our confidence. If your sleeping has not improved in the past few weeks, and you have followed the recommendations in this book carefully, then consider reviewing your sleep medication with your GP. If your sleep is still poor, the medication doesn't appear to be having the desired effect. That is reason enough to consider your reasons for taking it. If you have lost confidence in your ability to sleep, and you feel reliant on sleep medication, this reliance will interfere with your recovery.

If your insomnia is improving as a result of the changes you have been making, this might be a good time to discuss your options with your GP.

RELIANCE ON ALCOHOL AS A SLEEP AID

Are you taking alcohol regularly (some or most nights) in order to help you sleep? If your sleep is now improving, consider cutting down on the alcohol over the coming weeks. With the changes you have put in place, you may no longer need alcohol to help you fall asleep. If you do cut down, do so gradually.

If you are using alcohol each night, and your sleep is not improving, there could be several reasons for this. Some of these reasons may relate to other factors, as we'll see later in this section, and some could relate to alcohol specifically. Alcohol can be helpful as an aid to *falling* asleep. Unfortunately, alcohol frequently leads to shallow and disturbed sleep. As the alcohol in your bloodstream is broken down, the body starts to experience withdrawal symptoms. These withdrawal symptoms then interfere with sleep.

After alcohol consumption, a person may experience less REM sleep in the first half of the night. As a result, the second half of the night may feature excessive REM sleep, leading to vivid dreams or nightmares. Alcohol can help a person relax, and get to sleep more easily, but it does not lead to good-quality sleep. It leads to dehydration, excessive sweating and an over-relaxing of the upper airways. This is problematic because snoring or sleep apnoea then worsens, further interfering with sleep.

Finally, if you are waking up in the night needing to use the toilet, alcohol consumption might be the culprit. So, if your sleep diary tells you that you are getting to sleep well enough, but your sleep is being interrupted by periods of wakefulness, or if you are scoring your sleep as consistently poor, alcohol consumption before bed is likely to be a factor.

MY BEDTIME IS FREQUENTLY TOO LATE

We put in place a golden rule: never go to bed before your preferred bedtime, and only go to bed when you feel sleepy. If you are consistently going to bed in the early hours, there could be several causes. Are you getting up at a consistent time? Is that time early enough? A consistent, early rising time is vital because it promotes your body's drive to sleep.

Is your bedroom comfortable, quiet and dark? We unconsciously avoid things we dislike, often without realizing we are doing so. Go to your bedroom now, stand in the middle of the room, and take a good minute or so to decide how you really feel about it. Is it welcoming or unsatisfactory?

Another common reason for staying up late is feeling too alert. Ideally, you're not drinking caffeinated drinks beyond 3 p.m. in the afternoon, and (if you are a smoker) you're not smoking just before bed. If either of these things is problematic, use the exercise later in this chapter to help.

If coffee or cigarettes isn't the problem, try taking a shower or bath, or going for a walk in the evening. Remember to consider whether you find yourself too hot or cold at night when showering. If you are watching TV, surfing the internet, reading books or working until late on some nights, you would benefit from a period where you avoid these activities for a good 30–60 minutes before bed. Instead, try practising the exercises in this book.

Insight – Tai chi and yoga

There are many relaxing activities to choose from to help you unwind in the evening. Tai chi and yoga both come highly recommended for relaxation purposes, and they give other benefits as well. Both are easy to learn, either by going to a local class or from a DVD. These gentle forms of exercise help because they are comprehensive: they relax the body, relax the mind and relax the breath. Our thoughts, our feelings, our breath and sleep are inextricably linked.

Tai chi and yoga may also help if you're feeling anxious before bedtime. Even if you are sceptical, why not give one of them a try?

Staying up late could indicate a fear-based reluctance to go to bed. The *fast phobia cure* in Chapter 6 will help. Other sources of anxiety include worrying about day-to-day matters, events or problems that we just can't seem to stop thinking about. The exercises to deal with worrying thoughts (also in Chapter 6) can help you with this.

How is your day-to-day schedule? Is it regular, or irregular? Keeping a regular time for rising (and seeking out daylight on rising), breakfast, work, exercise, eating and socializing will help to set your body clock for earlier sleep. Consider changing your day-to-day routine if it is excessively disorganized.

CUT DOWN ON THE CAFFEINE

Have a go

▶ If consuming caffeinated drinks beyond 3 p.m. is a problem, this exercise will help.
▶ Use it when it is needed.
▶ It is straightforward and takes only 1 minute.

1 When you start to think about caffeinated drinks in the afternoon, what thoughts and feelings occur? If required, write them down. You may have mental pictures; for example, a steaming cup of coffee, or an image of yourself enjoying your drink. You may have a voice in your mind that tells you, *'Coffee would be good!'* It is likely that you'll feel some sense of desire or craving.

2 Take any images and squash them down in your mind, so they become small. Then, make them black-and-white. If a mental voice is talking about coffee, imagine that voice becoming quiet, like a whisper.

3 What would you prefer? Some people get used to herbal teas, and even begin to enjoy them! Water comes highly recommended for a variety of reasons. It is best to avoid sugary fizzy drinks, even decaffeinated ones. Instead, fruit juice, particularly mixed with water, might be a better idea.

4 Make a new mental movie that comes in two parts: a) you're enjoying the non-caffeinated drink, smiling, and then b) you're retiring to bed tonight and falling asleep. Think to yourself, in a calm but firm voice, *'I choose sleep, because sleep is better!'*

5 At that point, hold the mental movie described in Step 4 in your mind, and think about how much you really want to improve your sleep. You'll start to feel a sense of desire; spin those feelings around (see Chapter 3) so they become stronger, while repeating Step 4 several times.

This exercise is very simple, but it works. You're building a new association between desire at that moment, and sleep. Make Step 4 look enjoyable. You don't want your facial expression to be, '*Urrgh!*' You want it to be, '*Aahh!*'

CUT DOWN ON THE CIGARETTES

> ## Have a go
> ▶ If smoking a cigarette before bed is difficult to stop, try this simple exercise as and when you need it.
> ▶ It takes only 1 minute.
>
> 1 Typically, your last cigarette before bed will be smoked in the same place and most likely at night-time. This is a trigger. Make a mental movie of where you'd be, and what you'd see at that point as you got up to have a cigarette.
> 2 Take this mental movie, make it black-and-white, dissociated (so you can see yourself in the picture), and then make it smaller and smaller.
> 3 Then, replace that mental movie with a new movie, a big, colourful picture of yourself shrugging off any desire to smoke, and instead choosing to go to bed, and then sleep.
> 4 At this point, in your mind, tell yourself, '*I want that!*' As you picture yourself shrugging off any cravings for the usual last cigarette, remember how much you prefer going to sleep instead.
> 5 Repeat this exercise a good few times. You will start to feel differently about the need for that last cigarette before bed.

Although smokers find smoking relaxing, nicotine is a stimulant. Try not to smoke for that last hour before bed. Instead, make your last cigarette an hour or so before bed.

IT IS TAKING TOO LONG TO FALL ASLEEP

If it seems like you are taking forever to get to sleep, there are several things that are worth looking at. Again, check caffeine consumption and make sure it is not interfering with your sleep. Are you sticking to the rule where you spend no longer than 20 minutes trying to get to sleep? It pays to be honest with yourself here. Spending longer than 20 minutes in bed awake will make sleep more difficult. Be strict with yourself on this rule; it is a key recommendation that will help.

Staying awake in bed for longer than 20 minutes means you are not feeling drowsy enough to sleep. The exercises in Chapter 7 will help, providing you use them! Reading through them doesn't help; practising them does. Using the *progressive muscular relaxation* exercise in bed, followed by the exercise to *feel drowsy at bedtime* and then the *guided imagery* exercise, each night, will help in the vast majority of cases.

It is easy for us to lose confidence in our sleep. Negative, limiting beliefs interfere with our efforts to overcome insomnia. If you feel that you are unable to fall asleep easily, take a look at the exercise to *change limiting beliefs* in Chapter 7, and use it on this specific negative belief.

If your mind starts racing when you try to get to sleep, the best advice is to get up, and use the appropriate exercises in Chapter 6. Lying in bed worrying will only make things worse. Getting up and doing something constructive will make things better. It might not feel that way at the time, but persist with this behaviour. It will pay off.

I AM NOT USING THE NLP EXERCISES

Sometimes, we fear change. Change can mean the unknown. A fear of change, failure or the unknown can inhibit us from doing those things that we know will be of benefit. The exercises in this book require practice, and at first they can seem difficult. It can be awkward to try each one out, having to refer constantly to the step-by-step instructions. Visualizing requires focus and attention. Often our minds wander or the images disappear.

The exercises in this book are incredibly powerful, providing you practise. If you are not sure where to start, practise the *progressive muscular relaxation* exercise, combined with the exercise to *make your inner voice sleepy*. Practising those two exercises frequently should help you make some headway, and your confidence will grow.

The more you practise the exercises in this book, the better results you will get. It is simply cause and effect.

I AM HAVING DIFFICULTY IN STAYING ASLEEP

Are you still waking in the night? If so, look at your sleeping environment. Is it noisy or too light? Too hot or too cold? Is your bed comfortable? If you share your bed, does your partner snore or have sleeping difficulties of their own? Is alcohol or anxiety a factor? The recommendations given earlier in this chapter can help.

If you do wake in the night, are you finding it easy to get back to sleep? Check the *Length of time spent trying to get back to sleep* row, and the *Did I use the NLP exercises?* row in your sleep diary. Remember to try the exercise to *make your inner voice sleepy*, the *progressive muscular relaxation* exercise, the exercise to *feel drowsy at bedtime*, and the *guided imagery* exercise (or all four), to help you get back to sleep. If you do not fall back to sleep within 20 minutes or so, be strict with yourself and get out of bed for a spell. You might feel tired, and it might seem counter-intuitive, but getting up will make a positive difference to your sleeping patterns in the long term. Instead of just lying there, get up and practise with the exercises from Chapters 6 and 7.

I AM WAKING UP TOO EARLY

If you are waking very early, follow the recommendations above. After 20 minutes or so, if you cannot get back to sleep, try getting up and doing something relaxing instead. You may feel tired that day, but lying in bed awake will also leave you feeling tired, *and* it will promote further sleeplessness. On those occasions when you do get up early, avoid compensating by going to bed early on the following night. Wait until your preferred bedtime, even if you feel sleepy that evening.

Do you believe that waking up too early is always going to happen? If so, use the exercise to *change limiting beliefs* in Chapter 7, focusing on the idea that you will always wake up too early. Changing that belief can only help.

I AM SOMETIMES WAKING UP LATER THAN PLANNED OR I AM SPENDING TOO MUCH TIME IN BED AFTER WAKING

Sticking to a set rising time can be difficult at first, particularly if you're struggling to get to sleep at night. Upon waking, even without sleep difficulties, most people feel drowsy or tired for the first 30 minutes or so. Also, our beds can feel very comfortable when compared with the harsh reality of getting up in the morning! Some people feel like they don't have very much to get up for. These factors combined can make it difficult to spring out of bed at the start of a new day.

An irregular rising time causes many problems. The body's drive to sleep becomes weak, as does our body clock. People with insomnia have an erratic body clock anyway, and an irregular rising time further weakens an already fragile system. Sticking to the rule about getting out of bed early is key to beating insomnia. Try the following visualization exercise when you're in bed at night. As well as this exercise, consider the following:

Make sure that you need to get out of bed to switch off your alarm; jump straight into the shower after switching off your alarm (and filling in your sleep diary!).

Have ingredients for your favourite breakfast, laid out the night before, and know that you're going to make it for yourself.

If you have a family pet, go and play with it.

Have your favourite tea or coffee in the house.

Enlist the (gentle) help of a friend or your partner.

Ideally you will keep your typical getting-up time consistent throughout the week, including weekends. If there has to be a deviation at weekends, make your rising time no more than 60–90 minutes later than normal.

GET OUT OF BED IN THE MORNING

Have a go
- ▶ This simple exercise can help people get out of bed more easily.
- ▶ It is best to use it when you are in bed, having completed the *progressive muscular relaxation* exercise in Chapter 7.
- ▶ It only takes 1 minute, and is very straightforward.

1 After completing the *progressive muscular relaxation* exercise, imagine lying in bed, asleep, the following morning. Make this a clear mental movie. Imagine a clock in the corner of the screen, ticking over to your desired rising time.
2 As the clock ticks over to your desired rising time, picture yourself waking up, stretching, maybe looking a little sleepy, but steadily rising from bed, and padding across your bedroom to switch off your alarm.
3 As you watch yourself rising, tell yourself, '*I want to get out of bed at [your preferred time]!*'

4 Repeat Steps 1–3 about three times. As you play this movie in your mind, get a sense of expectation, of belief, that this will happen in the morning. Then, move on to a nice, relaxing guided visualization, as detailed in Chapter 7.

This simple exercise is designed to programme your mind with what you'd like to occur, and at what time. According to Albert Einstein, your imagination is your preview of life's coming attractions. We can utilize this to our advantage.

I STILL FEEL TIRED DURING THE DAY

If your sleep diary indicates that you have achieved a fuller, deeper, more consistent sleep each night, and you are still feeling fatigued, or sleepy, during the day, then try making your bedtime earlier by 30 minutes for a week or so. After seven days, if you are still feeling fatigued during the day, make your bedtime earlier still by another 30 minutes. This gradual change to your bedtime is best implemented when the other recommendations in this book are in place. Making this change will increase the amount of sleep you get, and you should begin to feel less fatigued. Feeling consistently tired during the day can be a sign of sleep deprivation.

We often scapegoat our lack of sleep as being the main culprit for tiredness, but that is not always the case. There could be many reasons why you are not feeling great during the daytime. For example, there might be problems with your diet, dehydration or stress. Perhaps you have a different type of sleep disorder. If you increase your sleep by an hour or so, gradually, but find that your sense of tiredness is not improving, consult your GP for further advice.

MY QUALITY OF SLEEP STILL FEELS CONSISTENTLY POOR

Are you giving the quality of your sleep a consistently poor rating? If so, look at the ease with which you are falling asleep (or not, as the case may be), whether you are waking during the night, and whether you are sleeping until the desired time. If your sleep diary indicates that you are experiencing fewer problems and getting more quality sleep, your rating of your sleep should improve accordingly. What criteria are you using to judge your sleep? It should be the factors in the sleep diary, rather than how tired you feel during the day.

Perhaps you are sleeping better, but still feel tired. See the section above for more information on what to do about that.

If your sleep is still light or fractured, then try setting an earlier rising time; this will give your body a greater window of opportunity to build a stronger sleep drive during the day.

You might believe you will always experience poor-quality sleep. If so, employ the exercise to *change limiting beliefs* in Chapter 7, using a mental movie of having poor sleep. The belief that you will only ever have poor-quality sleep makes no sense when looked at rationally. People overcome insomnia all the time.

Putting these changes together

At this point it is likely that you will have implemented some of the recommendations in this book really well, and some not so well. That is to be expected; the point of this chapter is to help you troubleshoot any remaining difficulties and fine-tune the programme to your needs.

GENERAL RECOMMENDATIONS TO HELP TROUBLESHOOT YOUR SLEEP

Here is a summary of factors, guidelines and recommendations that will help fine-tune your sleep.

- ▶ Make your bedroom a comfortable place that you enjoy being in.
- ▶ Use your bedroom only for sleeping, reading this book or having sex.
- ▶ Set a regular time to get out of bed, and stick to it no matter how much or little sleep you get.
- ▶ Get out of bed no more than 10 minutes after you awake.
- ▶ Go to bed no earlier than your usual bedtime (even if you feel very sleepy).
- ▶ Go to bed only when you are sleepy.
- ▶ Spend no more than 20 minutes trying to get to sleep or trying to get back to sleep.
- ▶ Refrain from napping.
- ▶ Don't consume caffeinated drinks after 3 p.m.
- ▶ Avoid drinking alcohol as a sleep aid.
- ▶ Cut out that last cigarette before bed.

If you're struggling to get to sleep, pay particular attention to:

▶ Allowing yourself a spell of relaxing activity before bed.
▶ Your ability to overcome anxieties.
▶ Your ability to relax.
▶ Using your bedroom for activities other than sleeping.
▶ Your beliefs about your ability to sleep.
▶ Setting an earlier rise time in order to increase your sleep drive.
▶ Reducing caffeine and nicotine further.
▶ Matters to do with children or chronic pain (see Chapter 10).

If you're struggling to stay asleep, pay particular attention to:

▶ Making sure that your bedroom is dark, quiet, the right temperature and comfortable.
▶ Avoiding late-night alcohol and nicotine consumption.
▶ Dealing with anxieties and stresses in life.
▶ Using the appropriate relaxation exercises to try to get back to sleep.
▶ Making sure you get up if you cannot get back to sleep.
▶ Setting an earlier rise time in order to increase your sleep drive.
▶ Again, matters to do with children or chronic pain.

By using the information contained in your sleep diary, you can be much more specific when identifying the problems you face with insomnia. Whether the problem is getting to sleep, waking frequently or waking too early, you now have clear steps to take in order to resolve the problem.

Using this troubleshooting guide, pinpoint the next change that would help towards overcoming any remaining difficulties with sleep. Implement just one change at a time, consistently, for seven days or so.

There are many reasons why it can be difficult to implement an extensive programme such as this, especially from a book. As we have said throughout, learning happens best by acquiring small chunks of information, and applying it gradually. If you start with one small change and build on that, things will happen gradually; you just have to make a start and keep going.

In the next chapter we will look at special circumstances that can also feed into insomnia, such as dreams and nightmares, or chronic pain. We'll then look to the future: beyond insomnia, and a life of freedom.

10 TIPS FOR SUCCESS

1 Your sleep diary provides you with a rich source of data. By spending 10–20 minutes or so analysing your sleep diary, you'll be able to pick out trends, patterns and problem areas.

2 Alcohol consumed before bed is likely to disturb your sleep in the middle of the night. It can lead to fractured sleep, nightmares, waking in the night, dehydration and excessive snoring.

3 If you are frequently going to bed very late or taking too long to sleep, check the time you rise from bed each morning. Your sleeping environment, stimulants (such as caffeine), your ability to relax and anxiety are likely causes.

4 When struggling to get to sleep, remember to practise the exercises to *combat anxiety* (Chapter 6) and *promote relaxation* (Chapter 7). Negative beliefs also interfere with getting to sleep easily. The exercise to *change limiting beliefs* in Chapter 8 can help.

5 If you are having problems with waking during the night, or you are waking too early in the morning, consider whether your sleeping environment, alcohol consumption, anxiety or limiting beliefs are factors.

6 If you wake too early, the best thing to do is get up and practise the exercises in this book. You may feel tired for the rest of the day, but you avoid making your insomnia worse by staying in bed.

7 It is important that you rise each morning at the same (relatively early) time. If this is proving difficult, use the exercise to *get out of bed in the morning* and have the comfort of a nice shower, your favourite breakfast, or some quality time with your family or pets waiting for you.

8 If you still feel tired during the day, and your sleep has significantly improved, then go to bed 30 minutes earlier, and see if the tiredness improves. If there is no improvement, consider other causes of tiredness, such as chronic stress or a different type of sleeping disorder. It would be worth contacting your GP to discuss this.

9 If you are still rating the quality of your sleep as consistently poor, and yet your sleep diary indicates improvements, then consider the criteria you are using to judge your sleep. It should relate to the sleep itself, and not whether you still feel tired.

10 It is likely that you have found some of the changes in this book straightforward, but that others require more work. Use the troubleshooting guide in this chapter to iron out any remaining difficulties you have.

HOW AM I GETTING ON?

▶ *Have you spent 20 minutes or so going through your sleep diary looking for trends, patterns and problems?*
▶ *Have you reviewed the troubleshooting guide to find specific solutions to problems you might be having at the moment?*
▶ *If required, have you tried the exercises to help you stop drinking coffee or smoking cigarettes after certain times?*
▶ *Have you used the exercise to get out of bed in the morning?*
▶ *Have you understood what you need to do next to further improve your sleep?*

By this point we should have a fairly good implementation of the recommendations in this book. There will be room for improvement, and that is to be expected. The best advice now is to keep going. Use your sleep diary to pinpoint whatever problem areas exist, and follow the recommendations in this chapter to take things on to the next level.

Change happens gradually. You can add to what you've achieved so far by reviewing previous chapters and retrying certain recommendations again. It's like putting up a tent; at first it's just a collection of rods, cloth, string and pegs. Once the framework is in place, everything else makes more and more sense.

In the next chapter, we'll look at those special circumstances that can interfere with sleep.

10

Choosing freedom

In this chapter you will learn:
- *how to interpret your dreams and nightmares*
- *how to help kids sleep better*
- *how to use self-hypnosis to ease pain*
- *how to get the most out of this book.*

> *The universe is change; our life is what our thoughts make it.*
>
> Marcus Aurelius

In this final chapter we are going to explore some outstanding matters. We will look at dreams and nightmares, helping children sleep better, self-hypnosis and pain, and finally try to overcome any difficulties with making the changes recommended in this book.

Dreams and nightmares

Our sleep can be disturbed by dreams and nightmares. People who suffer with insomnia tend towards light and fractured sleep, which can lead to vivid dreaming experiences. Such experiences then further interfere with our sleep, particularly when it comes to nightmares.

Dreams are more than just random brain activity; they can contain messages that we can learn to understand. These messages are not found so much in the individual, symbolic elements of the dream, but rather in the emotional experience. It is the theme, not the detail, that is important.

For example, let's say a person has a recurring dream of visiting a castle with her husband, who is wearing an unusual pair of sunglasses. It's a place she's never been to before, and she is wearing a red dress that she once used to own. It is hot, sunny and she is happy. Suddenly, there is a crowd of people, seemingly from nowhere. She loses her husband in the crowd and becomes increasingly anxious as she tries to catch up with him. Despite struggling through the crowd, he is always just out of reach.

What is the message in this dream? Is it that she wants to visit a castle? Is it that she loved her red dress? Is it that she feels she is losing touch with her husband? In fact, these details are not particularly relevant. Dream diaries might point to the symbolism of castles or husbands and suggest a universal meaning, but this is overly simplistic. There is a far simpler, and more reliable, process for decoding our dreams.

DECODE YOUR DREAMS AND NIGHTMARES

Have a go

▶ This exercise can take anything from 5 to 10 minutes.
▶ Take a good step back from the details of your dream when ascertaining the theme. The obvious answer is not always the right answer.

1 First, ignore the specific, and distracting, details (the castle, the dress, the sunglasses): *concentrate on the emotions present in the dream at the time*. So, in our example, at first she felt happy, and then panicky and frustrated.

2 The second step is to look at the abstract dynamic present in the dream. What is actually happening, when you strip away the detail? What is the theme? In our example, the theme is one of sudden change for the worse. In her dream she went from happy to anxious and frustrated, because things (the crowd) were getting in between her and where she wanted to be (by her husband's side). Can you pick this abstract theme from the details? The castle, the crowds, the husband are not relevant. If anything, these elements exist in order to create the drama, the change from happy to anxious.

3 The third step is to ask yourself, '*What does this dream have to do with my life right now?*' The answer to this question might be clear or it might be obscure. For the woman in our example, circumstances had changed at work. She had a new boss who had made several changes to her way of working:

> changes she didn't like. Her experience of work had changed from being comfortable and happy, to one where she felt like things were getting in her way. She was fighting against this, but wasn't making any progress, and felt like she was being left behind.

So the meaning of the dream, most likely, had little to do with her husband, castles, dresses and the like. Her problems at work were *mirrored* in the dream. If you are troubled by a recurrent dream, it is well worth looking at it with the above steps in mind. Ignore the details; it is the emotions, and the theme, that are important. It can take a little time to discern the theme of a dream, but with practice you'll soon get the hang of it.

Insight – working with dreams

Sometimes, once you have recognized the message(s) present in a dream, you might then think, 'Well, so what? What can I do with this information?' It is not always the case that we can act on these messages. Often, however, once you get to the bottom of a dream, and its message, the dream tends not to recur and sleep therefore improves.

Dreams are easily forgotten. Even after a minute or so, they can be lost. If dreams play a part in your insomnia, keep a notebook and pen by your bed, and write down the details on waking.

Recording and decoding your dreams can improve your understanding of your hopes, your fears and your feelings about your life. With this better understanding, people feel more at ease with themselves; better sleep often follows.

Sleeplessness in children

Children have different sleep requirements from adults. Teenagers, for example, are known to have a more owlish body clock than adults, preferring to stay up late and get up late. This circadian rhythm-based tendency is typical among young people, and can be difficult for their parents to understand.

Younger children can also struggle with sleeplessness, as of course can babies (as any stressed-out parent will tell you!). However, there are things that can be done.

BABIES

Even at a couple of months old, babies can learn good sleeping habits. As a baby's body clock starts developing after six weeks, it pays to put these good habits in place as soon as possible.

We learned in Chapter 1 that our body clock is strengthened by having regular times for going to sleep, waking up, eating, socializing and the like. The same is true for babies. By setting a regular time each day for getting up, feeding times, bathing, going out and getting to sleep at night, this routine will lead to good sleeping habits. For some babies, it can take longer than others to learn, so you should persevere with this routine, even if it doesn't seem to be working. It just takes a little time.

Establishing a bedtime routine for your baby also helps. Each evening, carry out the same steps in the same order; for example, bathing, changing clothes, feeding, a relaxing cuddle and then laying your baby down for sleep. This lets your baby know when it is time to sleep, and sleep will become associated with the end of the routine. If your baby wakes in the night, following the same routine helps because, over time, your baby has associated the end of this routine with sleep.

Babies should be encouraged to fall asleep alone (known as *self-soothing*). If your baby cries when you put them down for sleep, aim to wait for a few minutes before attending to them. Some babies typically cry when they fall asleep, for example.

Just as with adults (who are overgrown babies, after all), exposure to daylight will help set your baby's body clock. In the morning hours, try to interact with your baby and teach them that daylight means being awake. At night-time, the opposite is true: be calmer, quieter, interact with your baby less and keep the bedroom dark, comfortable and quiet.

Babies, like all children, enjoy relaxing contact before sleep. Before putting your baby to bed, pay them some gentle, relaxed attention, and then let them settle in peace, alone, for the night.

TODDLERS AND SCHOOL-AGED CHILDREN

With toddlers and school-aged children, the advice relating to a regular daily schedule, a soothing evening routine and being able to self-sooth, also hold true. The main problem children of this age tend to experience relates to settling. It can take a while for young children to settle down to sleep, and during this period of restlessness they may demand your attention.

There are several things to consider here. First, there is no point sending your child to sleep if they are not tired. If your young child is frequently not tired at their preferred bedtime, then consider whether they are getting too much daytime sleep. If you try to send your child to sleep when they are simply not tired, you'll have a rebellion on your hands.

Insight – children form associations too

Bedtime needs to be a relaxing experience. Using bedtime as a punishment, or punishing your child for not going to bed, is one of the biggest mistakes you can make as a parent. From what we've learned together about forming associations, it seems obvious that the last thing you need is for your child to associate bedtime with punishment. This will only make them much more reluctant to go to bed.

Instead, bedtimes should be associated with *attention that has limits*. Rules around bedtime need to be enforced consistently, and delaying tactics should be ignored. Instead, offer to reward your child with an entertaining (and relaxing) story. Children love personal attention. Use this fact to make bedtime a special time that they enjoy.

Some time after putting your child to bed or during the night, you might find that they cry out for your attention. This can be a difficult thing to deal with. As parents, we want to reassure ourselves that our children are all right, and we can feel incredibly guilty if they seem upset. However, if you attend to your child at these times, you are rewarding them (with attention), which makes such behaviour more likely in future.

In such circumstances, either do not go to check on your child, or if that is too strict for you, check on them before calmly, gently and politely asking them to go back to sleep. Then leave the room, with absolutely no further interaction at that time. Your child will learn that such cries for attention are not going to get the results they desire, and will learn to self-soothe instead.

With children of this age, consistency is key. Remember to stick to the same evening routine. Make your own state relaxed, with a soft and gentle voice, and be calm and gentle as you remind them that it is time for sleep. Then, after they are ready for bed, take some time and read them a bedtime story. Read for the same length of time each night. Remember, if you are soft, gentle and relaxed at this time, they will take this as a cue to be relaxed too.

Have you been practising with the *guided imagery* exercise in Chapter 7? By the time children are of school age, they tend to respond very well to guided imagery if you can hold their attention. After reading your child a story, why not ask them to close their eyes, and have them imagine they are riding on a magic carpet, playing an amazing game of football, watching their favourite TV programme, or whatever you know they would love to imagine. Engage all of their senses: what they can see, what they can feel, what they can hear. Focus their awareness inwards, and suggest to your child that soon *their imagination will turn into a really pleasant dream.*

Self-hypnosis for better sleep

Self-hypnosis is an excellent way of combating stress. It is simple, relaxing and a good way of preparing yourself for sleep. Once in self-hypnosis, auto-suggestion can be used to ease problems with IBS, pain, asthma, migraine and panic disorders.

We are going to look at a standard self-hypnosis induction, followed by suggestions for pain relief. This process should be used only for chronic pain, never for acute pain, or where the basis for the pain remains undiagnosed. Pain is an important matter, and the use of self-hypnosis for pain relief should be discussed with your GP first.

Self-hypnosis is widely considered to be safe and beneficial. However, you should seek medical advice before using self-hypnosis, particularly if you are experiencing mental health issues (for example, depression, bipolar disorder or schizophrenia). In some cases, for example, where a person is very introspective or has a tendency towards depression, then medical advice should also be sought first.

Have a go

▶ This exercise takes around 5–10 minutes.

▶ It works best after the *progressive muscular relaxation* exercise from Chapter 7.

▶ After completing the self-hypnosis induction, use the *guided imagery* exercise, also from Chapter 7.

▶ It is best to use this exercise in bed before you go to sleep.

▶ This exercise involves a lot of talking: for some it works best when speaking out loud; for others, speaking internally is best (particularly if you share a bed with a partner).

▶ In our example we are going to focus on pain relief; however, you can also use this simply for better sleep, for less anxiety or to feel refreshed in the morning and so on.

1 Once you have completed the *progressive muscular relaxation* exercise, tell yourself that you are going to go into self-hypnosis and then fall asleep.

2 Then, state the goal you would like to achieve while in self-hypnosis. For example, '*I am entering self-hypnosis to ease the pain of my arthritis and sleep comfortably. My unconscious mind will make all of the changes and adjustments it needs to help me.*' (Always include the line about the unconscious mind at the end.)

3 In your mind's eye, imagine being in a relaxing place. It could be on a beach, in a forest, a summer terrace or in a comfortable room by an open fire. Wherever you would like to be. (In our example, we will focus on being on a beach.)

4 Using your drowsy voice (see Chapter 7), slowly note something you can see in your mind's eye, '*I am looking at a blue sky.*' Then note something you can hear in your imagination, '*I can hear the sound of the sea.*' Then note something you can feel in your imagination, '*I can feel the sun against my skin.*'

5 Then repeat Step 4 but think of two things you can see, two things you can hear and two things you can feel: '*I can see the sea stretching out to the horizon... I can see a seagull gliding across the sky... I can hear the sound of my own breathing... I can hear a child's laughter in the distance... I can feel sand beneath my toes... I can feel a gentle breeze in the air.*'

6 Then repeat Step 4 again, this time thinking of three things you can see, three things you can hear and three things you can feel. Each item you observe in your imagination must be different, so really absorb yourself in the visualization; what details can you pick out?

7 Now that you're relaxed and absorbed in the visualization, imagine that your pain is a fuzzy glow in your body, and give it a colour. Use your imagination to make the colour drain, so it fades. Imagine you can reach into the fuzzy glow and soothe it, so it becomes smaller, diffuse and weaker. This is similar to the *spinning feelings* exercise in Chapter 3; gently ease the feeling of pain so it moves backwards on itself. This will cause the pain to ebb away.

8 As you carry out the visualization in Step 7, say to yourself, '*This pain is easing away to be replaced with relief and relaxation.*' Come up with your own suggestions, focusing on the word 'relief'. How does it feel when a painkiller kicks in? Use your memory of that experience and incorporate it into the visualization.

Although this exercise is very simple, it does require practice. It can be used at any time. Simply modify Steps 1 and 2:

1 Once you have completed the *progressive muscular relaxation* exercise, tell yourself that you are going to go into self-hypnosis for 10 minutes or so.

2 Then state the goal you would like to achieve while in self-hypnosis. For example, '*I am entering self-hypnosis to ease the pain of my arthritis and when I come out of hypnosis, I will be pain-free. My unconscious mind will make all of the changes and adjustments it needs to help me.*'

If you're going to use this exercise during the daytime, it is best not to do it where you might fall asleep! Only ever use self-hypnosis when it is safe to relax completely; never use it when driving or operating machinery.

Practising this exercise for a week or so will be of great benefit. Not only does it aid sleep, it can be used to help you make changes in your life: increasing confidence, motivation or determination, for example.

Problems with implementing the recommendations in this book

Making changes in our lives can be difficult. We've discussed previously how fear can inhibit action, even beneficial action. Problems with low motivation or feeling overwhelmed can also hinder our progress. Sometimes conflicts within the home, such as a lack of understanding from our partner, make things difficult. Each of these factors can lead to a despondency that stops us from improving our lives. How many self-help books end up discarded and forgotten?

Making changes in our lives requires focus, determination and persistence. Life can be viewed as a mechanical system where each and every action (or inaction) counts towards something.

- ▶ You have dishes to wash? If you do the washing up, that action will count towards something: in this case a clean kitchen. If you leave the washing up, that inaction will also count towards something: in this case a dirty kitchen.
- ▶ You have a report to write? Write it, and your action will have counted. Avoid writing it, and your inaction will have also counted.
- ▶ You have a friendship you want to strengthen and enjoy? If you behave like a good friend, the friendship will grow. If you avoid behaving like a good friend, the friendship will suffer.

Everything counts towards something. In the same vein, accumulation comes from repetition. Imagine a person, about to go on a diet in order to lose some weight, resolving to eat a healthy salad for the next 100 days. Over the coming 100 days, they then eat salad on 90 of those days. A good effort; they have accumulated 90 days' worth of healthy eating. As a result, it is likely that their goal of shedding some weight will be achieved.

Imagine a second person with a similar goal and a similar plan. During their 100-day period, salad is eaten on just 15 of those days. Unfortunately, only a small amount of healthy eating has been accumulated, and as a result it is likely that their goal of shedding some weight will be missed.

So when we repeat an action, we accumulate. The opposite is true when we repeat an inaction: we'll have an *absence* of accumulation. When you think of your efforts to implement the recommendations in this book, what have you accumulated? Although simple, many of the recommendations in this book require *repetition* in order to work.

▶ You have insomnia to overcome? If you use the tools presented in this book, your actions will count towards improved sleep. Avoid using the tools in this book, and your inaction will count towards a failure to improve your sleep.

If you have been using this book for the past three weeks or so, what repetitious action have you tried, and what has it accumulated? If you filled in your sleep diary on most mornings, that action will have accumulated towards pinpointing problems with your sleep. If you used the relaxation exercises on most nights, that action will have accumulated two things: a greater ability to relax, and more hours spent asleep. If you followed the recommendation to rise at a fixed time each morning, you will have accumulated a greater drive to sleep during that period. Permanent change is frequently dependent on accumulation via repetition.

Let's take a look at some typical obstacles for making changes, so that we might overcome them.

FEAR OF FAILURE OR CHANGE

A common obstacle to changing things in life is the inertia created by irrational fears. What makes a fear irrational? Imagine, if at the age of ten, a child were to forget his lines in a school play. In that dreadful moment, with all eyes on him, panic sets in and eventually he runs from the stage, crying. This event is not going to be forgotten by the brain. Rather, it will be remembered as something to avoid in future. Some years later, an adult now, this person is asked to be best man at his friend's wedding. At first elated, he then thinks of the speech he'll have to give, and dread sets in. At this point, the brain is recalling (unconsciously) the fear and upset of the childhood experience, and fears that the adult experience will be the same. This is a generalization, and it has formed a limitation in his mind.

We have all tried to make changes in the past and failed miserably. You may have attempted to overcome your insomnia several times before reading this book. Unsuccessful prior attempts to change condition people to avoid trying again. With this in mind, it is recommended that you start with the simple changes. You cannot fail at readying your bedroom for better sleep, providing you keep going. Making all of the required changes, at most, would take a day or so.

148

From there, focus on getting up at a consistent, relatively early hour, and staying up each night until it is your bedtime and you feel sleepy. While doing that, focus on learning the relaxation exercises. These three changes can make all the difference for many people. They are relatively easy to implement. As you read this, remember how much you desired better sleep when you purchased this book. That desire means something. Your life will be better when you act on it.

LOW MOTIVATION

When suffering from insomnia, problems with low motivation can be difficult to overcome. People with insomnia tend to be tired, and sometimes insomnia coexists with other difficulties, such as depression or anxiety. Motivation can be difficult to come by.

What is motivation? In this context, we are referring to the motivation to do something. Motivation, or a lack of motivation, is a multifaceted experience encompassing our conditioned associations, our habits, our beliefs, our fears, our thoughts, our emotional state, our desire, our experience of expectation, pressure and inertia, and our behaviours! That's quite a list: it is not simply a case of, '*Stop being lazy!*' People who struggle with low motivation tend to procrastinate.

Procrastination is the irrational act of putting something off, even though it would benefit us to act. Everybody has been guilty of procrastination at some point in their lives. The effects of long-term procrastination can be debilitating. Interestingly, a major cause of procrastination is the fear of change or failure we mentioned earlier.

The recommendation to keep it simple is applicable in this case as well. Concentrate on making your bedroom an ideal sleeping environment, getting out of bed consistently (at a relatively early time) and using the relaxation exercises. If procrastination is a problem, in Chapter 5 there is an exercise to *become more determined* that you can put to good effect.

Insight – enlisting the help of others

Public expectation also helps people overcome problems with low motivation. Is there anyone you can enlist to help? Family? Your partner? Perhaps a close friend may be willing to harangue you each morning until you get out of bed! This wouldn't need to go on for ever, just long enough to establish the habit of rising earlier. Similarly, if you tell people in the office that you're not going to drink coffee after 3 p.m. you're more likely to succeed. Enlist the help of family, friends and colleagues. You're much more likely to succeed than if you attempt things on your own.

FEELING OVERWHELMED

Tackling insomnia is often a straightforward case of addressing your sleep environment, adhering to sleep hygiene recommendations, learning how to relax and quieten your mind, and regaining trust in your ability to sleep. However, if it really were that simple, then you'd have done that already, right?

There are a lot of recommendations in this book. NLP is easy to do, but it can be overwhelming at first. The recommendations in this book, although straightforward, need practice. The chapters in this book are ordered in a specific way. They will guide you through a series of small, incremental exercises that bring about the change you are looking for: to find sleep more easily.

Feeling overwhelmed can also be a disguised fear of failure or change. Without realizing it, we start to become anxious and think less clearly. We don't know where we're up to and worry about getting things wrong. Impatience can also be a problem: trying too much, too soon. Instead, as above, focus on making your bedroom a comfortable place that you only use for sleep, get up at a fixed time and only go to bed when sleepy. From there, practise with the relaxation exercises. Take each step slowly, concentrating on just small changes that happen one at a time.

LACK OF SUPPORT FROM FAMILY MEMBERS

It is not uncommon for there to be tension in situations where one person has insomnia, and their partner or family members do not. This tension can arise from a lack of understanding or clear communication. As a result, there can be sulking, arguments, sleeping in different rooms and even divorce. Does it need to be this way?

Sometimes, the source of the tension is solely to do with insomnia. In such cases, the non-sufferer might find it difficult to accept their partner's problems. Unless he or she has studied the causes of insomnia they might dismiss it, instead imagining that their partner just needs to try harder to get to sleep. When changes are proposed, removing the TV or attempting to get out of bed earlier, this lack of understanding can cause resentment, arguments and unhappiness.

Such problems with understanding and communication are rarely one-way. The insomnia sufferer may react angrily to this lack of understanding: arguments escalate, people become defensive and positions become entrenched.

In such cases the only solution is clear communication. Better communication aimed at a deeper understanding, followed by a practical arrangement that will benefit you both. Aim to be pragmatic, solution-focused and, most importantly of all, non-accusatory. Accusations will just sabotage your efforts to implement the changes in this book, and should be avoided at all costs.

Sometimes, arguments about insomnia, and the recommendations in this book, are simply another reason to bicker. In a relationship that has broader difficulties, a lack of care, trust or understanding, simply ask yourself, 'Is it any wonder I can't sleep?' Many people struggle with insomnia because they know there are significant, unaddressed problems in their lives. If your relationship with your partner is frequently full of arguments and misunderstandings, then addressing the broader issues might help.

One step would be to talk with your partner honestly. Lay your cards on the table and explain what it is you want and need in your life. Taking such a step depends entirely on your judgement. What response are you likely to receive? Again, be reasonable. Relationships do require compromise. However, if you're in a relationship that is frequently causing you heartache and misery, then this situation is most probably contributing to your insomnia.

By now, you should have implemented some of the changes recommended in this book. Some recommendations, although they might prove beneficial, will have been discarded or glossed over completely. To overcome any remaining difficulties with insomnia, what is the next, best step to take? Which chapter would you benefit from re-reading?

The reality is that some of the people who read this book will not engage with the exercises in any meaningful way. Instead of trying to learn from it, the book will be read passively, not taken in and put to one side. The result? Sleeplessness will persist, and an opportunity to change has been missed. Don't be one of those people. Complete what you have begun, and you will soon see yourself as a person who can sleep easily.

If you have completed the exercises in this book, and your sleep is improving, the following, simple exercise will help you to keep it going.

Have a go

- ▶ This exercise takes around 1 minute.
- ▶ It works best after the *progressive muscular relaxation* exercise from Chapter 7.
- ▶ It is best to use this exercise when your sleep is improving, and you want to further cement the gains you have made.
1 Once you have completed the *progressive muscular relaxation* exercise, imagine yourself some three months from now.
2 See yourself looking healthy, happy and relaxed. Make this image look believable, by giving it the same look and feel as your picture of belief (see Chapter 3). Watch as you go about your business.
3 Fast forward a little, and see yourself going to bed at night, and easily falling asleep. Watch yourself for 10 seconds or so, sleeping well without waking, until the morning.
4 As morning breaks, watch yourself get up, and take a shower. See yourself looking refreshed and relaxed.
5 State to yourself, 'Look, I am a good sleeper!' As you say this, really believe it.
6 Watch yourself doing the things you'll be doing, a few months from now, with this new-found vitality and energy.
7 Repeat this exercise several times, and make it feel good!

It won't take long for you to see yourself as a good sleeper, and our journey together is almost complete.

In conclusion

What is really happening in your life right now? As far as we know, we have but one life to live. One life to achieve our goals and live for our values. Is your insomnia making life difficult, or is a difficult life causing your insomnia?

Whatever your frustrations, your pains or your fears, you can choose to live a life of freedom. The exercises in this book will help you overcome insomnia if you spend a month or two putting the recommendations into action. Beyond sleeplessness, what else can you achieve? What goals would enable you to step beyond limitation and pain, and lead a different kind of life?

Learning how to overcome insomnia is about learning to overcome obstacles; learning to change things in your life for the better. By making progress with this you are, in fact, learning how to take control. Use this book to change the way you think, and everything else can change as well.

Practise, practise and then practise again. The more you use the visualization exercises the better your results will be. Learn to control your inner voice, your inner images and the emotions that you feel. Fear, limitation and restriction are experiences you have with your mind, first and foremost.

You are not immune to difficulties in life; serious things can happen. In fact, the only thing we can predict in life is unpredictability. However, realize that you are not helpless, nor is life hopeless. To step beyond limitations such as sleeplessness takes courage and determination. If given enough time and attention, this book will have equipped you, to some extent, with tools that will open your mind. Now focus, and take a huge stride forward.

10 TIPS FOR SUCCESS

1 People who suffer with insomnia tend towards light and fractured sleep, which can then lead to vivid dreaming experiences.

2 Dreams are more than just random brain activity; they can contain messages for us to decode and understand.

3 The messages in dreams are not to be found in the detail; instead, look at the emotional content and the abstract theme of the dream.

4 If dreams play a part in your insomnia, keep a notebook and pen by your bed and write down the details on waking. Understanding your dreams can lead to better sleep.

5 To help babies and children sleep, set a regular time each day for getting up, eating, bathing, going out, and getting to sleep at night. This routine will lead to good sleeping habits.

6 Establishing a bedtime routine for your children also helps. Each evening, carry out the same steps in the same order. Babies and children will come to understand that the end of this routine is a time to sleep. Consistency is key.

7 Self-hypnosis is safe and beneficial. Use the *self-hypnosis* exercise in this chapter to help with pain relief, anxiety, motivation problems and more. (If you have experienced mental health issues at any stage in your life, speak to your GP first).

8 Problems with a fear of failure, feeling overwhelmed or low motivation can be overcome by starting off small and making little advances. Begin by addressing your sleeping environment, as per Chapter 4, and then look to implement a consistent, relatively early rising time each day. From there, practise with the relaxation exercises in Chapter 7.

9 Difficulties in relationships can sometimes be addressed with better communication. If your partner seems unsupportive,

it could be due to a lack of understanding rather than a lack of caring. Aim to be pragmatic, solution-focused and non-accusatory. If things still don't improve after that, then honestly look at the broader health of your relationship.

10 The sad truth is many people will give up before completing this book. Don't be one of them. Finish what you have started, and your chances of success are as high as they could be. You *can* get to sleep at night. All you need to do is make a start and then keep going.

HOW AM I GETTING ON?

▶ *Have you put a notepad and pen by the side of your bed to record the details of your dreams? If vivid dreams play a part in your insomnia, have you tried the exercise to* decode your dreams and nightmares?

▶ *If you have children, have you started putting in place a regular daily routine and a regular evening routine to help them sleep more easily?*

▶ *Have you tried the* self-hypnosis *exercise? Practise it regularly for best results.*

▶ *How does the information relating to a fear of failure or change, or feeling overwhelmed, relate to your own experiences with this book? Have you understood fully that your destiny is in your hands?*

A freedom from sleeplessness and insomnia awaits. All you need to do now is keep going. You can have the sleep you want if you work towards it, and the recommendations in this book can help. The most important thing to remember is that you're not trying to get to sleep, you're reconnecting with your own innate ability to sleep. Even if you feel you have lost that ability (you haven't), your mind and body can be reconnected with it. Every action counts. Good luck!

Index